MW01107628

MY NAME IS
ALYSA

MY NAME IS ALYSA

*Medical Journal,
Spiritual Way*

Kathy Evernham

LUTHERS
New Smyrna Beach
F L O R I D A

FIRST EDITION
Copyright © 2002 by Kathy Evernham
ALL RIGHTS RESERVED

Published by
LUTHERS PUBLISHING
1009 North Dixie Freeway
New Smyrna Beach, FL 32169-6221
www.lutherspublishing.com

PRINTED IN THE UNITED STATES OF AMERICA

Jacket design by Mike Halen

JOY COMES IN THE MORNING. Words by William J. and Gloria Gaither.
Music by William J. Gaither. Copyright © 1974 Gaither Music Company ASCAP.
All rights controlled by Gaither Copyright Management. Used by permission.

Excerpt from COLD SASSY TREE by Olive Ann Burns.
Copyright © 1984 by Olive Ann Burns. Reprinted by permission
of the Houghton Mifflin Company. All rights reserved.

Scripture taken from the HOLY BIBLE, NEW INTERNATIONAL VERSION®
Copyright 1973, 1978, 1984 by International Bible Society
Used by permission of Zondervan Publishing House. All rights reserved.
The "NIV" and "New International Version" trademarks are registered in the
Unitied States Patent and Trademark Office by the International Bible Society.
Use of either trademark requires the permission of the International Bible Society.

LIBRARY OF CONGRESS
CATALOGING-IN-PUBLICATION DATA
Evernham, Kathy, 1942–
My name is Alysa: medical journal, spiritual way
Kathy Evernham.—1st ed.
p.   cm.
ISBN 1-877633-62-3 (pbk.)
1. Conselyea, Alysa—Health.
2. Encephalitis—Patients—Michigan—Detroit—Biography.
I. Title.

RC390.C66 E95 2002
362.1'96832'0092—dc21   2002016121
[B]

ACKNOWLEDGMENTS

It is with great respect that I thank my parents for their love and encouragement throughout my life. Their keen interest in reading, words, and writing instilled in me a foundation for creative expression. Even the word games played during long car trips piqued my delight in the nuances of words and their meanings.

I thank my husband, Tom, who patiently waited to use the computer and finally gave up and bought a second computer for himself. His excitement and support for my writing of this book were paramount.

Kisses, hugs, money or whatever he wants to my son, Jeff, for reformatting the first twelve chapters into a computer style that efficiently facilitated the word processing of the entire manuscript. I promise to read the Microsoft Word manual—one of these days. Thanks also to Donna, Jeff's wife, who gave early feedback and critique that helped clarify and direct the story.

Blessings to son Kevin whose faith in my success continued to buoy my spirits. I thank his wife, Christa, for explaining her registered nursing knowledge and procedures in terms my layman's brain could understand. Technical thanks also go to Dr. Don Stogsdill for further clarification of medical apparatus and procedure.

Dr. Jeff Benjamin's contribution in reading, editing and scrutinizing the entire manuscript is deeply appreciated. Without his help, the work would have lost its medical credibility.

I thank my pharmacist niece, Joelle Evernham Lynch, for the correct spellings of the drugs mentioned and the purposes for which they were dispensed.

I reserve my most heartfelt thanks to my sister, Carole June Greene, whose English teacher/writer background served her superbly as my editor. As each chapter was faxed hundreds of miles away, she applied her crisp, to-the-point corrections and shaped the readability and coherence of the manuscript. After my whining, she learned that my performance improved when she threw me a few bones—like "good sentence." Having a Jewish editor enhance and hone a Christian book took a great deal of courage and sisterly love. May God give her the glory; especially since she isn't getting paid.

I cannot thank the Conselyeas enough for their candor and willingness to re-live and share their personal pain. Their foresight to keep journals plus their intact memories of all the events helped the book to write itself. May they know an abundance of God's blessings.

FOREWORD

Louis E. Rentz, D.O., F.A.C.N
President and CEO
Michigan Institute for Neurological Disorders

I have been practicing in the field of medical Neurology for 30 years. I am certified in Neurology by two American Specialty Boards, and have been a clinical professor of Neurology at Wayne State University and Michigan State University-College of Osteopathic Medicine. For much of this time, I have been director of a residency-training program in Neurology, a member of the Specialty Board, and for the past 15 years the Executive Director of the American College of Neuropsychiatrists, an osteopathic Specialty organization for both Neurology and Psychiatry.

I briefly note my training and qualifications only to highlight the fact that in all my experience, I have not encountered a case similar to that of Alysa Conselyea: a case with which you will become extremely familiar as you read this intriguing and fascinating account.

Infections of the nervous system come in a variety of types. The most common is that of meningitis. The meninges are both hard and soft tissue coverings that surround the brain and spinal cord and contain the spinal fluid. "Meningitis" is used to describe irritation of this brain-covering material. It usually consists of two types: viral and bacterial. Viral meningitis produces a headache and inflammation but no actual bacterial or fungal growth. It can be mild. It is seen sporadically and sometimes seasonally. In general, it produces headaches, fever, and minor confusion and is almost always self-limiting as it clears with little or no neurologic sequelae.

The second type, "Bacterial meningitis," is an infection of the brain by bacteria, generally of either meningococcal or streptococcal type. It can be very severe and is the type of meningitis that gains attention when someone becomes extremely ill or dies.

Encephalitis refers to inflammation of the functioning brain cells themselves rather than the covering of the brain. A virus enters the cellular structure and produces severe disturbance in function. It generates abnormal function of cells resulting in a wide variety of neurologic symptoms including seizures, abnormal movements, loss of memory, personality change and hallucinations as well as loss of balance and motor control. It can be mild and transient or it can be severe, progressive, catastrophic and fatal. This is the form of infection we believe Alysa contracted.

With the exception of a few specific infections, there is no known treatment for the majority of cases of viral encephalitis. Most of the time, we cannot make a specific viral diagnosis. Spinal fluid may only be suggestive of mild inflammation because, again, the inflammation is in the brain rather than around it as happens in meningitis.

As you read *My Name Is Alysa*, you will become well aware why the physicians involved in Alysa's care are often asked and ask themselves, whether her case represents a miraculous cure.

The answer, I believe, is that a series of minor and major miracles are involved in Alysa's odyssey. One miracle exists in the love and concern of the physicians, technicians, nurses, and therapists who apply extreme concern, care and devotion to prevent numerous complications from ensuing in a case of prolonged, severe illness. Many complications do transpire—phlebitis, pneumonia and urinary tract infections. But the care Alysa receives prevents many others—bedsores, pressure sores, and traumatic injuries.

The ultimate miracle is a testament to the faith and belief of Alysa's family and friends and to the faith and good will of individuals of multiple religious beliefs—Catholic, Protestant and Jew alike. As you read this remarkable story, you will decide for yourself the authenticity of miracles.

Dedicated
to my grandchildren
Kyle, Ryan, Chloe,
Alexa, Julia and Kassidy.
Like the tiny mustard seed,
may you grow in faith
and reap great results
for God's kingdom.

CHAPTER ONE

Anguishing in the emergency room of a suburban Detroit hospital, Linda Conselyea realized a mother's worst nightmare: her daughter Alysa was slowly slipping into an abyss of unreality. Waiting in the corridor for the social worker's return, Linda tried to control her rampant emotions. While Dave Conselyea puzzled over their predicament, Linda's thoughts hop-scotched over her daughter's actions of the past week.

*   *   *   *   *

"Grandma, I don't feel good. I've got a headache, I think," Alysa had announced Monday as she came home from the beauty salon where she worked.

"What do you mean, you think you have a headache? Don't you know?" Sylvia Rivers asked her granddaughter.

"No, I've never had one before."

"Here, I'll get you a few Tylenol. Take them and lie down. You should feel better in a little while," Sylvia said as she put her palm on Alysa's forehead.

Alysa went to the bedroom that had been hers for the past year. She had lived with Grandma and Grandpa Rivers in Royal Oak since she started attending the nearby David Presley College of Beauty in 1995. After graduating from beauty school, she began her apprenticeship at the Bardha Salon, located in

1

Birmingham, which was also in the area. It was a convenient arrangement for her.

Could her headache be the result of the chemicals at the salon? Perhaps a short nap would do the trick. But no. More symptoms appeared later that afternoon.

"Sean! Billy! Would you two just be quiet or go downstairs where you won't bother anyone!" Alysa sternly reprimanded her two young cousins, Billy, 11, and Sean, 9. The Rivers watched their daughter Vicki's children after school every day. The boys loved Alysa, who was usually affectionate and loving with them.

"Jeez. What's wrong with her?" Billy asked Grandma as he rolled his eyes toward Alysa.

"I really don't know, Billy. Alysa never raises her voice at you boys. She isn't herself today," Grandma replied. To Alysa she said, "Honey, what's wrong?"

Alysa burst into tears and wailed, "I just don't know!"

Automatically, Sylvia again felt her granddaughter's forehead. "I think you might have a slight fever. How do you feel?"

Rubbing the tears from her eyes, Alysa said, "I've got spots in front of my eyes. And I feel sick to my stomach."

But after supper, Alysa bounced back and seemed fine. She laughed and played games with her cousins and helped them with their homework. In fact, her behavior was so silly and childish that Billy looked at Alysa and asked, "Are you on drugs or something?"

The Rivers' small house was overrun with people. It was week two of their son Marc and his family's visit from California. With all of the people under foot, Alysa's slight complaints soon were overlooked. Linda and Dave, Alysa's parents, added to the fray when they came each day to spend time with everyone.

Alysa took her mother aside that night to speak to her confidentially.

"Mom, I had a massage a week ago today. It felt wonderful, but I didn't like what the therapist did afterwards. When the woman was finished, she did this weird thing with her hands, like a trance, over my body. She placed them just above my pelvis, then my stomach, then my chest and last, my head. She called each point a 'chakra' and said it balanced the energy flow in my body. I didn't like it. It was creepy. Do you think that could have

2

affected me?"

"I really don't think so, Alysa, but why don't we pray about it?"

They held hands and Linda prayed for her daughter's unease to go away. Alysa seemed content after that.

Alysa had attended a hair show in East Lansing the day before. As a Redken trainee, she had been asked to participate. At the last moment, she had been reluctant to go.

Ransacking through her drawers, her purses and other stacks of feminine clutter, Alysa had yelled, "Where's my money? I can't find my money? Where on earth is it?"

She had saved money for her trip to East Lansing for several weeks and now had misplaced it. She threw herself on the bed and sobbed.

Sylvia, hating to see Alysa so upset, went into the room.

"Lysa, Honey, don't worry about the money. I can give you whatever money you need. Here, take this. You can always pay me back when you find your money."

In a surprisingly child-like voice, Alysa said, "Oh. Grandma, you are so wonderful. I just love you." She hugged her grand-mother around the neck. Then in a split second, Alysa abruptly changed her mind and said, "I don't want to go! I won't go!"

"But, Honey, you've been wanting to do this for a long time. You told me you hoped to become a Redken representative," Sylvia said, confused over Alysa's sudden change of heart.

Somewhat chastened, Alysa responded, "Okay, I'm almost packed. Thank you for the money. I will pay you back."

Late that Saturday afternoon Alysa had driven the seventy-five-mile trip to East Lansing in her black Chevy Beretta. The show was successful and Alysa must have made a good impression, because the Redken leader asked her to do another show in the fall. Alysa would be unable to keep that appointment.

She had shared a hotel room with Marie, another Redken trainee from a different salon. Early on Monday morning, Marie awakened and was startled when she saw Alysa in the bed next to her.

"Alysa! What's the matter? You're soaking wet. Your hair is dripping. How did you get all wet? Did you take a shower and go back to bed?"

Drowsy and hesitatingly, Alysa had replied, "No, I haven't been out of bed. I don't know what's wrong. I feel strange."

"Strange? What do you mean, strange?" Marie had asked.

"Like I'm not me. Like I've been somewhere. Oh, I'm cold," she added, shivering.

Later, the incident forgotten, they both packed up their gear and headed to their cars.

"Hey, Lysa, you take care, y'hear?"

"Sure, Marie. You, too. It was good getting to know you. God bless you," Alysa said in parting. She had to be at the salon in Birmingham for afternoon appointments. But that was the day that she had come home early with her first headache.

On Tuesday she met with her boyfriend, Ken, for lunch. They missed each other over the weekend. But after only an hour, Alysa returned to Sylvia's. She sat in her car, by the curb, crying, then entered the house and hurried toward her room.

Her grandmother looked up as she rushed past. "Alysa, you look pale. Is something wrong?" Sylvia asked.

"Why is everyone asking what's wrong all the time? I don't know what's wrong!" she answered, stomping into her room and slamming the door.

Sylvia was stunned. This strange-acting person was not her loving, happy-go-lucky Alysa.

The next morning, Wednesday, Linda received a call from a distraught Alysa.

Using a childish, brokenhearted tone of voice, Alysa said, "Mommy, I woke up last night and couldn't remember the words to 'Jesus Loves Me.' Grandma sat on the couch with me and helped me sing it. I forgot the words." Switching to her normal voice, Alysa forlornly said, "And I can't sleep. It is so black when I close my eyes. I feel like my soul is dead."

"I'll be there in a little while. We'll go to your dad's office and we'll pray about this."

Although for Linda, prayer was a normal approach to problems, she still felt a shiver of fear climb her spine. She picked up Alysa and drove to Dave's real estate office. Dave saw Linda and Lysa get out of the car, and again was struck by their startling resemblance. They could be sisters…twins, even. He met them at the door.

4

"Hi! How are my two favorite girls?" His exuberance faded. He could tell by the look on Linda's face that this was a serious visit, so he took them into his conference room where they could be undisturbed. Alysa described how she felt the night before. The family spent time talking to each other and more time praying together.

"I feel so much better now," Alysa said afterwards.

Dave grabbed his sport coat off the coat rack. "Why don't we go and get some lunch?" They went to Bill Knapps and ordered their favorite things. No one ate much, and Dave and Linda closely watched their troubled daughter.

Thursday at work, Alysa started to cry. Mrs. Baker, the shop manager, took Alysa into the hair color mixing room. "Alysa, why are you crying? What's wrong?" she asked solicitously.

"I don't know. I can't get a grip. I can't seem to stop crying," she replied between sobs.

"Well, if you can't pull yourself together, I'm going to have to send you home." Unconvincingly, Lysa said, "Okay, I'm going to try." But Alysa couldn't control her crying and was soon driving home to Grandma's.

Linda was there when Alysa arrived. Her blotchy eyes and red nose immediately revealed that she had been crying. Linda put her arms around her daughter and comforted her.

"Alysa, are you okay? What happened? Is it Ken?"

"Oh, Mom, I don't know. For some reason, I can't stop crying. It's like something bad happened in Lansing," she said.

"Bad? Where? To you? What happened? Tell me." Linda nearly panicked.

"I wish I could. I don't remember. I just know that something bad happened."

"Alysa, I don't understand how you can know something happened, but not know what it is. Are you afraid to tell me? Did you see something? Did someone touch you? Were you molested?" Linda asked, getting more frantic.

In her now familiar child-like voice, Alysa said, "Mommy, I just don't remember." She started to cry again.

These unpredictable mood swings were unnerving to Linda. When Alysa quieted, she asked her daughter, "Lys, I don't know what is happening with you, but I think it would be good if the

5

elders prayed for you. What do you think?"

"I would really, really appreciate that," she said.

Linda called the Faith Baptist office, thanking the Lord that it was still office hours. "Hi, Carol, this is Linda Conselyea. Alysa is under some kind of stress and maybe even a spiritual battle. I'd like for the elders to pray over her," she told the pastor's wife.

Not daunted by the request, Carol replied, "Jim isn't available, but I can round up several of the elders. Is 6:30 okay with you?"

"That would be an answer to prayer," Linda replied.

Early that evening Linda thought she witnessed a change in Alysa's countenance as these churchmen prayed for Alysa's deliverance from this unknown illness.

In bed that night, Dave and Linda discussed this new revelation of something "bad" happening in Lansing.

"What do you think might have happened?" Dave asked Linda.

"Do you suppose she could have been raped?" Linda questioned in return.

"Oh, good Lord, I hope not. Maybe it was drugs. Somebody could have given her drugs without her knowing it," he said.

"How can we find out? She seems to have blocked out whatever happened."

Dave responded, "I guess we could call the salon and ask who the Redken guy was and contact him. He might know something."

"Yes, we could," Linda said. "She certainly has been acting funny since the trip to Lansing. I don't understand this little-girl voice. And sometimes she's singing and dancing around. It's like her hormones are wacky."

They repeated what little they knew and came to no conclusion.

"Oh, don't forget, Dave. We're supposed to meet everyone at "Ping Ons" in Sterling Heights at 7:00 tomorrow night. Ken is going to pick up Alysa."

Her name was the last word uttered that night and was the bridge into Linda and Dave's subconscious entrance into sleep.

The Friday night dinner was to be a gala farewell for Marc, Diane and their young sons. Marc often teased his favorite niece, but his actions were subdued on this occasion. He had regarded her quizzically as she seemed unusually remote. Alysa became nauseated at the restaurant and Ken took her home to Grandma Rivers. Linda had wanted to go to her mom's to check on Alysa when she and Dave left the restaurant, but she had to go home to work on a wedding cake order.

Linda scraped the white frosting off the counter but ignored what had smeared onto her apron. Her workspace was adequate for the task at hand, but the wedding cake stretched the tiny kitchen to its limits. The different flavored layers were strewn around the swirled 1960s style Formica countertop waiting for her attention. She gave the chocolate walnut layer its coating and set it next to the already frosted banana and lemon layers. As she picked up the raspberry cheesecake layer, the phone rang. She glanced at the clock wondering who would be calling her at 11:00 at night. Dave was down in the family room sleeping in front of the TV. When Dave didn't answer the phone, Linda wiped her hands on a linen towel and grabbed the portable. It was Alysa.

"Hi, Mommy. I just had to talk to you," Alysa said in her little-girl voice.

Still puzzled by her daughter's childlike voice, Linda inquired, "How are you feeling now, Alysa?"

Next, in an adult voice, Alysa said emphatically, "Mom, I've got it! I know what God wants me to do. I have to tell Billy and Sean about Jesus. They have to go to church. They need to know about the Lord."

My poor daughter, Linda thought. What is going on with her? Giddy one moment, serious the next. She behaves like her normal 21-year-old self and then becomes a little girl calling Dave Daddy and me Mommy. It is absolutely bizarre.

"Honey," Linda said, "Did you get some rest? Are you still sick at your stomach?"

"Yeah, Ken left and I slept for a little while, but I started having nightmares. Mommy, I'm scared."

"Why don't you try to get some more sleep and I'll come over tomorrow after I deliver the cake. Lysa, I'm sorry I can't be there with you, Sweetie."

"That's okay. I'll see you tomorrow. G'night."

Linda turned back to the cake with a heavy heart. She couldn't and wouldn't disappoint her friend and the 200 people at the wedding, but she really wanted to be with Alysa. She spent the wee morning hours shaping and placing the white frosting roses around the cake. While she worked, she constantly prayed for Alysa.

The next morning Linda had to force herself out of bed. She dragged into the shower to wake herself up. Dave had brewed the coffee much earlier before he left for his office to do some Saturday morning catching up. The wedding cake had to be delivered by 11:00 and she planned to leave the house by 9:00. She put the fresh flowers on the cake and entwined the ivy around the tiered layers. It looked beautiful. The real trick was going to be transporting it over the back gravel roads to get to Addison Oaks Country Club in Rochester. She had already called the county to find the best route that would keep her on primary roads. Oakland County, Michigan, one of the richest counties in the United States, still had 850 miles of unpaved roads. She arrived at the reception site by 10:30. The cake had made the trip unscathed. To her surprise, there was Dave.

"Dave, what are you doing here?" she asked, knowing it was quite a drive for him.

"I had the camera at the office and I knew you'd want a picture of the cake, so I came over to get some pictures of it."

"I don't know why I am surprised. You're so thoughtful. My head isn't on anything except Alysa."

Linda got the cake set up, he took some shots, and then they kissed good-bye.

"I'm going over to Mother's. I'll be there all day. Marc and Diane leave around 4:00."

"Okay, when I'm finished at the office, I'll be over. Tell Lysa I love her."

Linda bounded into her mom's house, anxious to see how Alysa was doing. Alysa was downstairs watching a movie with her young cousins. Diane, Linda's sister-in-law, found that moment to speak to Linda privately.

"You know, if I didn't know Alysa any better, I'd think she were pregnant. At least, that's how she's been acting these past few days. She's moody and cranky and then she just oozes with affection. I sure hope she's better soon."

"Thanks Diane, I hope so, too," Linda said.

The California Rivers contingent got off to the airport on time.

8

Linda remained with Alysa. Ken and Alysa were going to a party that night and Alysa had volunteered to bring a cake. Hoping that baking skills were hereditary, Ken had thought that he and Lysa would bake a cake for the party plus make special cakes for their mothers for Mother's Day. Alysa said no.

"Mom, can you bake the cake for me?" Alysa asked. "I don't have the energy to do it. I'm going to take a nap. I feel so out of it. I can't function."

Doing something would keep Linda busy, so she was glad to have the distraction. She baked the cake and was decorating it in her professional style when Alysa came into the kitchen.

"Oh, Mommy," she sang as she danced around. "I can't believe you're doing this for me. You are the best. Thank you, thank you, thank you!" She hugged her mom and kissed her.

Ken and Alysa went to the party and presented the cake. Linda drove back home to Davisburg. But Lysa's mood changed and she wanted to go home. Later in the Rivers' basement family room, Sylvia and Andy Rivers and Ken and Alysa were watching a rented movie when Alysa spookily spoke out.

"I don't know where I am right now."

Sylvia reacted. "Alysa, Honey, you're at my house and we're in the basement."

"Oh," said Alysa.

This wasn't the first time that Alysa acted out of it. The night before when Ken brought her home from the restaurant, she ended their date with uncharacteristic abruptness.

"Ken, go home," she had ordered.

Ken, momentarily miffed at her rebuke, reminded himself that Alysa had been acting funny. Mature enough to not have hurt feelings, Ken shrugged his shoulders.

"Umm, okay. I'll call you in the morning. I want to discuss what we're going to do for Mother's Day on Sunday. It would be neat to surprise our moms." He intentionally leaned over to give her a kiss good night, but she had turned and left the room, apparently forgetting he was there.

CHAPTER TWO

May 12, 1996, was Mother's Day. Mother Nature greeted the day in her own perverse fashion: she chose to ignore the calendar. Although the sun shone brightly, the weather was freezing cold. Renegade clouds whisked by and shed tiny snow pellets upon the unsuspecting Michiganders.

On Sunday morning, Dave typically enjoyed his coffee out by the lake. Shivering, he strode along the shore and onto the dock. Hastily he returned to the warm house beating his arms with his hands trying not to drop his favorite mug, the one inscribed "Number One Dad."

"Man, is it ever cold out there!" he told Linda. "You had better wear your winter coat. I thought this was May."

Linda tidied their breakfast dishes. Before leaving for church, they spent a few moments in prayer, as they always did.

Jim Combs, the gregarious, uninhibited 38-year-old pastor, was in his usual good form. When he preached, the congregation never knew if he'd walk on the pews or run up and down the aisles. A real people-person, he just loved greeting his church family. He glad-handed and hugged members as they assembled. The growing Baptist church counted nearly 2,000 as members and he knew the names of most.

This day, he preached about mothers and their roles in God's family, their own families and in the community. Dry eyes were uncommon on most Sundays, and as he talked about his own mother, this Sunday was no exception.

Spiritually fed, Linda and Dave left church ready to kick back and enjoy the day with their families. They made a quick shopping stop so they could honor their own mothers. They went to the Canterbury Village Shops for items Linda had previously seen but not purchased. For Roselind, Dave's mom, they bought a "Welcome To My Garden" plaque, and for Sylvia, they got a verdis outdoor stand that said "Welcome."

"You've saved the day again, Honey," Dave said. "Mom'll just love it."

They were driving to his folks, the Conselyeas, first and then to Sylvia and Andy's to eat dinner and celebrate. The gifts were never opened.

Meanwhile in Royal Oak, Ken and Alysa had walked to a nearby park. Alysa was restless and Ken thought a change of scenery might help. They sat on the swings and gently pushed back and forth. Suddenly, with great urgency Alysa opened their conversation.

"Demons and the devil are after my family. I have to protect them. Ken, I want you to be saved," she added.

A lot to absorb at once, Ken ignored her first utterances and responded to the latter.

"Alysa, we've talked about this and if I do make that decision, it will be when I'm ready, not before," he told her earnestly.

"Right. We won't talk about it," she snapped.

Wanting to cajole her he said, "No. That's okay. We can talk about it. You just surprised me, out of the blue, so to speak."

"I want to go back, now," she said. They returned to the Rivers where Alysa became agitated and extremely talkative, a total switch from minutes before. Grandma Rivers was convinced that Alysa needed medical attention.

As Dave and Linda drove to the elder Conselyeas' home, Dave's cell phone rang. Normally calm, Sylvia was on the verge of hysteria.

"Alysa is worse. I think you've got to take her to the hospital right away!"

They had 15 minutes of the 25-minute drive yet to go. Linda called Dave's parents and cancelled their visit with a promise to call them later. They filled those minutes guessing, speculating and praying as they sped down I-75 to Royal Oak.

"Father, God, please protect my daughter," Linda prayed over and over. They ran into the Rivers' and found Alysa crouching on the sofa. She seemed disoriented, her mind not quite with it. She didn't respond to her parents' ministrations.

"Mom," Linda said, "I'm going to call our friend Dr. Dolven and ask his opinion."

Craig Dolven, a GP who had been in an auto accident, had personal experience with neurological situations. Louann, his wife, had become one of Linda's regular customers when she operated her candy shop in Clarkston.

Linda found the number and dialed the phone. Apologizing for calling Craig at home, Linda explained that their regular doctor was out of town and she needed immediate advice concerning Alysa. She explained the symptoms that Alysa had been exhibiting for the past few days.

"I think she needs to be evaluated," he urged. "You should take her to the emergency room right away."

The ride to Bellville Hospital* was quick. The emergency room was not crowded and, surprisingly, the Conselyeas did not have to wait long for Alysa's admittance. Dave filled out the necessary paperwork while Linda waited with Alysa in examination room number three.

A flashily-clad male nurse conducted the vitals assessment: blood pressure, pulse rate, temperature, heart and lung function. He had bleached blonde hair, painted fingernails and several pierced earrings...in his ears, at least. Alysa was in one of her talkative moods and they exchanged hair and nail techniques, topics familiar to her trade.

"I just love that color polish," Alysa said. "What is the name of it?"

He splayed his long nails in the air and said, "Oh, this color, Honey? I think it's called 'Romancing the Tone.' Isn't that a kick?"

*The names of all medical facilities and personnel have been changed for reasons of privacy. Any similarity is purely coincidental.

"And your hair, is that a high lift blonde or just straight bleach?"

"Little girl, there isn't anything straight about me."

Alysa found this statement hilariously funny and they both laughed at the joke.

Dave entered the area and was greeted by the child-like Alysa. "Hi, Daddy. I love you," she said. She put her arms around his waist and hung on.

"I love you, too, Sweetie."

In a nano-second, she changed and with growing emotion said, "I'm sooooooo concerned about Ken's salvation. I'm afraid he's going to die without Christ. And Billy and Sean. They never go to Sunday School and they don't know the Lord. I need to tell them. I just don't do it right," she said dejectedly with her head lowered.

"Don't worry about that right now. We'll talk about it later."

A physician entered the sheet-partitioned cubicle and introduced himself. "Hello, I'm Doctor Masters, the attending physician. What seems to be the problem here?" he said, directing his question to Alysa.

Alysa, hyper and disoriented, began a run-on monologue.

"I don't really know, for sure. You see, I've been having nightmares, and spots in front of my eyes. Oh, and headaches. And I've never had headaches before. And I'm not sure where I am and I cry for no reason and it could be from the massage when she introduced demons to me or maybe it was in East Lansing. And I've been sick to my stomach. I don't know."

With raised eyebrows, the doctor looked at Linda and then Dave for help in deciphering Alysa's words.

"She hasn't been herself recently, Doctor," Linda understated. "She has been behaving strangely for the past few days. She will be agitated and very talkative and then she becomes moody and withdrawn. She has had a slight fever and complains of headaches and spots in her eyes. At times she talks like a little girl, but most of the time she is completely normal. That's why it is so baffling."

"What does her reference to demons mean? And what about East Lansing?" he wanted to know.

"I don't know if those are relevant. She had a massage a couple weeks ago and Alysa was exposed to an eastern meditation technique that bothered her. We are Christians and don't condone what we consider an opening into unknown spirits. Anyway, I'm not sure that is important. But she has been worried that something bad happened in East Lansing when she was there for a hair show. She doesn't remember anything about that," Linda concluded.

The doctor ordered a blood work-up (a CBC), and a CAT scan. He turned back to the patient.

"Alysa, what day is it today?"

"It's Sunday, Mother's Day."

"Who's the president of the United States?"

"It's Clinton, unfortunately," said Alysa as she grinned.

"What is your full name?"

"Alysa Marie Conselyea."

"Have you been given or taken any drugs recently?" he interjected.

"Drugs? Me? Never! No, I'd never take any drugs!"

"Are you sure? What happened in East Lansing?"

Her face twisted with consternation, and she replied in a very soft voice, "I don't know. I just don't know."

The nurse returned to draw blood and then to take Alysa for her CAT scan. Linda and Dave talked in quiet voices in the not-so-private cubicle.

"There's a problem with insurance," he began. "Alysa doesn't have any and she isn't covered by our policies anymore. I guess that's something we hadn't considered. I feel just terrible about it."

"Oh, Dave. She has always been so healthy. I hadn't given it a thought, either. Maybe it won't be a problem. Let's pray about it." They joined hands and prayed for the situation at hand. They prayed to their Lord, the great Provider of everything his children need. They were calmed and comforted in the knowledge that God hears and answers their prayers.

Looking pale and vulnerable, Alysa was wheeled back into the room and helped back onto the examination bench. Becoming agitated, she demanded, "Mom, why did you bring me here?"

"Well, Lysa, you haven't been yourself lately. We thought you should be checked. Remember your headaches? And crying?"

In total denial, Alysa shouted, "No! I'm fine. I want to leave."

Dave responded, "Lys, Honey. Let's wait and find out what the doctor has to say, okay?"

"Okay," she flip-flopped.

Alysa fell asleep while they waited for results from the blood tests and the CAT scan. What seemed like eons later the doctor came in with the results. The blood test was negative for pregnancy, AIDS, and drugs. The CAT scan also showed nothing unusual.

"So, I'd like for you to talk with someone from Social Services. Perhaps we'll find some answers from that arena," he said. "Ms. Brandon would like to speak to Alysa alone. Could you step out into the waiting area? Or, if you'd like to go to the cafeteria, I can direct you."

"Uh, we'll just stay nearby, Doctor. Thank you," Dave said.

Linda and Dave found two ugly, uncomfortable, molded plastic hospital chairs in the drafty hallway and sat down. The chairs matched their feelings. "I don't like being excluded," Linda admitted.

"I agree. I don't see why we can't be in there with her. Why someone from Social Services? What does that mean?" Dave asked her.

"When I worked here, years ago, Social Services was just then becoming a big part of the hospital scene. They try to connect people with the right programs or facilities when they leave the hospital. They soothe the relatives of patients, and I guess they can help with a diagnosis. I don't know. We'll have to wait and see," Linda finished.

Ms. Brandon had asked Alysa many probing questions, and Alysa was losing her temper.

"I already answered that," Alysa snapped, exasperated. "I know what day it is."

"Where do you live?"

"I live with my grandparents in Royal Oak."

"Why do you live there and not with your parents?"

"Because it's close to school and work. My folks live way out in Davisburg."

"What symptoms have you been having?"

"Nothing. I'm fine. Now, can I go home?" Alysa said, not realizing her answer was not the truth.

Writing on her clipboard, Ms. Brandon told Alysa, "You just lie here and rest awhile. I'm going to talk to your parents now."

*   *   *   *   *

Ms. Brandon approached Linda and Dave and jolted Linda out of her recollections of the last week and back to the present time. The social worker was somewhat slovenly with her attire, Linda observed. She was unkempt, with her hair askew, and she wore no make-up. Her self-introduction contained no warmth.

"Mr. and Mrs. Conselyea, did I pronounce that correctly?"

"It's 'KON-sell-yay,'" Dave responded. She held out her hand.

"Marlene Brandon. Could we go over here? I'd like to discuss your daughter's case," she said, looking only at Linda.

"Apparently, the blood work revealed nothing. Nor did the CAT scan. I've talked to Alysa and it is evident that she is disturbed. I'd like to ask you a few questions. Mr. Conselyea, I see from the admission form that you are not Alysa's biological father?"

"No, I'm not. But I never think of myself as not being Lysa's father. She's my daughter, even if it is by adoption and not by blood," he insisted.

She turned to Linda. "Mrs. Conselyea, you are divorced, then." It was a statement, not a question.

"Yes, a long time ago. But what does that have to do with Alysa?"

"Children can develop psychological problems long after a troubling episode in their lives," she answered. "One never knows when unusual behavior will be manifested. Alysa said she does not live at home. Is there tension in your home?"

"Absolutely not!" Dave blurted. "We miss her tremendously. She's had transportation problems and it's a wonderful arrangement for her to be with her grandparents. They love having her, and it's convenient to her work. We still see her every other day, at least," he added.

"Do you think she has taken drugs?" Ms. Brandon asked.

Dave calmed down and said sincerely, "Look, Alysa is the perfect daughter. She's never done drugs. Oh, she's probably tried a beer once or twice, don't you think, Linda? Maybe she's tried a

16

cigarette, but I doubt it. She hates smoking. She's really a goody-two-shoes. She's a normal, happy kid. We just want to know what's wrong with her. If it will help, we'll tell you the far-fetched stuff Linda and I've been trying to figure out."

"Okay, please do," she said.

Approaching a path of no return, Dave began. "You will probably think I'm out of my mind, but Alysa may have had a paranormal experience. She had a massage and the therapist did a practice that some say is a form of demon worship. Now, Alysa is a strong Christian, and a Christian cannot be possessed. Having Christ in your life would protect you from demon possession. But, a Christian can be oppressed, rather, can be engaged in a spiritual battle. The devil already has the rest of the world, but he'd like to have the Christians most of all. So, anyway, we think there is a remote possibility that this massage affected Lysa's personality," he finished sheepishly.

Ms. Brandon had listened to this explanation with apparent incredulity. She made a few notations on her chart and asked, "What about East Lansing?"

Linda, also wanting to be helpful, without couching her words, answered.

"Lysa doesn't remember what, but she has said several times that something bad happened in East Lansing. We've thought of everything. Could she have been raped? Could someone have put drugs in her food? Or maybe she saw something terrible. We're just at a loss for what she meant."

Analyzing the records and considering the information from her interviews, the social worker wrote at the bottom of her report "Psychiatric treatment strongly recommended."

Only months later would Dave and Linda realize that their daughter's future medical care had been based on the diagnosis of a social worker. The head ER nurse at Bellville, a friend of Linda's, called to order a cake. Although she had not been on duty the day Alysa had been admitted to the ER, she had access to Alysa's charts, and in casual conversation she revealed the prejudicial analysis that stigmatized the diagnosis of Alysa's illness.

"You can go back in with your daughter now. The doctor will be in again to talk to you. Good-bye."

They walked back into the emergency room. "She's as friend-

17

ly as a snake," Dave said.

"A snake demonstrates more compassion than that woman," Linda commented.

They found Alysa awake and confused. "Why am I here? Let's go home."

"Alysa, as soon as we talk to the doctor, we'll be able to leave. That shouldn't be too much longer, Honey," Dave told her. But emergency room time creeps by slowly.

"I've got to call Sandy," Linda told Dave. "I'll be back in a few minutes."

Sandy was the mother of the groom at the wedding the night before. She was a Bible Study Fellowship lecturer and Linda was one of the children's leaders.

"Hello, Sandy? This is Linda."

"Linda, the cake was out of this world, everyone…."

"Sandy, I'm sorry to interrupt. We've brought Alysa to the emergency room today and we don't know what's wrong. We're waiting to hear from the doctor. I don't know what will happen next, so I'm not going to be able to be at the BSF leader's meeting tomorrow. Please have everyone pray for her."

"Oh, Linda, I'm so sorry. Of course, we'll put her on our prayer list. Keep me posted, okay?"

"I will, Sandy."

That was the first prayer list to record Alysa's name and situation. Eventually, there would be hundreds.

Two hours later Dr. Masters returned. "We haven't found anything medically wrong with your daughter," he said to the parents. "We think that maybe she is experiencing a psychological problem. We would suggest that she be examined and assessed by a psychologist or a psychiatrist. We've done all we can. I'm sorry I don't have a better answer for you," he added when he saw the looks of disbelief and rejection of his diagnosis. "I can give you a few names if you'd like."

"No, thanks. I know of some people I can call," Linda said. "Thank you, Doctor, for your help."

Dave shook the doctor's hand and then turned to his daughter. "It's over, Lys. We can leave now. I'm starved. What about you? Would you like to get something to eat? It's almost nine o'clock."

"Whatever," she replied, listlessly.

Alysa was dismissed. They walked through the waiting room to discover Ken and many of his relatives waiting anxiously. Ken's family had become quite attached to Alysa during the one-and-a-half years they had been dating. Alysa immediately went to Ken who gave her a big teddy bear hug.

"We've all been waiting for you. How ya' doing?"

"I'm tired," she said as Ken's mom, Linda Beaudoin, and his sisters, Kelly and Carrie Komisarz, anxiously gathered around her.

They shared their sympathy of her ordeal and said they were glad she was going home. Ken's family would offer tremendous support in the medical drama that was about to unfold and encompass their lives.

Dave, surprised by the crowd and feeling protective of his daughter, took her elbow and said to Ken, "We're going to go get a bite. No one has eaten. Do you want to join us?"

"Sure. Where are you going?"

"National Coney Island. It's close," Dave answered.

Wanting to lighten the mood, Linda and Dave did not let themselves think of the pronounced recommendation. They had barely started to eat when Alysa turned to her parents.

"Mommy and Daddy," she said in her little-girl voice, "Is it okay if Ken takes me home?"

"Sure, Honey. You've had quite a day. You go on home. Good night, Sweetie," said her dad.

Alysa walked to her mom and gave her a hug and a kiss, "G'night, Mommy."

And then to her dad, "G'night, Daddy."

"Good night, Lysa. We love you."

Linda and Dave drove home in silence, feeling drained.

19

CHAPTER THREE

Taking the social worker's recommendation to heart, Linda phoned some Christian psychiatrists the very next day. She spent the afternoon tracking down people who could help Alysa. An urgent call from Ken squeezed through.

That was the day that Alysa had a court appearance because of a recent auto accident. The girl who hit Alysa happened to have a father who was an attorney, and he was posturing in his own realm to have the case resolved in his daughter's favor. Ken brought Alysa to her dad's office so she could speak with their attorney, Mike McCulloch, whose office was in the same business complex.

Right away, Dave noticed Alysa's remoteness. Ralph Conselyea, Dave's 81-year-old dad, still loved going to work and contributing to the company. Ralph stretched out his arms expecting his usual hug and said, "Hi, Alysa. How's my girl?"

"Hello," was all Alysa said.

Surprised and a little hurt, Ralph dropped his arms.

Dave ushered Ken and Alysa into the conference room where Mike was waiting. "Alysa, the judge is going to ask you some questions and you need to be prepared," Mike instructed. "Now, what direction were you going?"

"I was going that way," Alysa answered, pointing off-handedly toward the windows.

Oh, oh, Dave thought. This is going to be trouble. All of Mike's questions were met with her distant, unfocused state. Losing patience, he dismissed her, "Okay, Alysa, you're off to see the judge."

She never made it to the courthouse.

*   *   *   *   *

"I'll never forget that day," said Ken. He had taken the afternoon off work to lend his moral support for her court hearing. "We met with Mr. McCulloch. He wasn't trying to put words in Alysa's mouth, but he was coaching her on how she should present her side. He'd tell her how to state it, and five minutes later, she wouldn't remember. She kept saying, 'I'm just not with it.' I was not looking forward to this ordeal."

"We were driving down Main Street in Royal Oak and Alysa was looking wide-eyed out my sunroof—like something had frightened her. Then she started convulsing. I was frantic! I pulled over to the side of the road and ran into a mechanic's shop. 'Quick, call 911, my girlfriend is having a seizure!' I went back to the car and was horrified to see that she was turning blue, drooling and had slipped into unconsciousness. I was afraid to touch her. It seemed like forever, but the EMS arrived in only five minutes. I ran back into the shop and called Linda. 'Alysa has had a seizure and the ambulance is taking her to Bellville,' I told her. As they took her from my car and put her on the gurney, she regained consciousness and became combative. 'Don't touch me! You're not going to take me anywhere! Ken, help me!' she shouted at them. It was pitiful! Then, she returned to a more normal state than I had witnessed for three days. I followed the ambulance in my car. When we arrived at the hospital, she was still calm and cooperative."

*   *   *   *   *

At the courthouse, Dave paced the corridor and repeatedly glanced at his watch. "Where on earth are they?" he asked the air. Ken and Alysa had been right behind him on his drive to the courthouse. He had been waiting for 45 minutes and the case had already been called.

"Excuse me, are you Mr. Conselyea?" a young woman asked.

21

"Yes," Dave hesitantly replied.

"There was a phone call from your wife. She said that your daughter has been taken to Bellville Hospital. She will meet you there."

The always-polite Dave left without a word of thank you to the messenger. Dear Lord, what now, he thought.

Alysa had been admitted to the eighth floor. She had overcome the first seizure but was now agitated and talkative. A blood test was the only test administered. Linda asked and was granted permission to stay throughout that first night. Sleep was non-existent as Alysa stayed awake most of the night.

Linda: "We were frantic to know what was wrong. I went into the room side bathroom, slid down the wall to my knees and cried to the Lord for his help and mercy. Words didn't come. I just offered my hurting soul and asked for his loving grace and his strength. I would always feel better after prayer. It was my salvation."

In casual conversation that night, a friend suggested to Dave that he might want to keep a journal to record the medicines as well as the doctors' diagnoses. Little did he know the number of entries they would record.

Tuesday, May 14, 1996
Day 2

* The doctors are stymied. More blood tests. Alysa getting more agitated. Ate a little breakfast. During the day she had second seizure. A bad one. Grandma Rivers, Linda, four nurses and myself present during this seizure. It took all of us to try to calm her down. Dr. Hanson tried to do a spinal tap, but said it was too difficult. Doctors talking about doing MRI. Dr. Conrad, resident psychologist, says could have been psychosomatic. I don't believe it.

Alysa was not as disoriented as the first night; instead she was energized. She was alert, wide-awake and strong. Angry, too. Valium, administered to try to quiet her, didn't work. Her behavior became even more bizarre. Dave spent that night with his daughter.

* Italicized words represent entries from journals kept throughout Alysa's illness by family and friends who stayed with her.

"I want out of here!" she screamed at her dad.

"No, you sit down right now."

"YOU sit down right now!" she shrieked.

Dave's journal noted that she was totally out of control. "Honey, you've just got to calm down," he said to non-listening ears.

Alysa paced the room all night. She had superhuman strength and stamina. "I can't get a grip," she kept saying.

"Where are you, Alysa?"

"I'm in Bellville Hospital."

Minutes passed and she turned to her dad and frantically asked, "Where am I?"

Next, standing on the bed, then jumping up and down, she said, "There's an aura around me." Wildly wind-milling her arms over her head, she said, "I'm God!"

"No, Honey, you're not God."

"Who are you?" she suddenly asked.

"I'm Dave, your dad, Alysa."

Rocking, she asked, "Who am I? I feel this presence. God is everywhere."

"Lys, we're going to get this worked out."

"Well, I know...I'm Satan."

"No, Honey, no." That's when Dave's charismatic background surfaced.

"I command you in the name of Jesus, with the blood of Jesus, to depart from this girl!" demanded Dave. He didn't know what else to do!

Alysa screamed at the top of her lungs. People stared. "Let me out! You can't keep me here." Then in a different, compassionate voice, "God loves that lady," pointing to the woman in the other bed.

"Shh, shh, Alysa."

Louder, and singsong, "God loooovves you!"

Dave didn't know whether to laugh or cry. It was funny, but it was horrible. All night long Alysa kept asking who am I? What day is it? Obviously, the Valium was not having a calming effect. "It was so scary. I didn't know why she was doing this. This is really unbelievable, I told myself. What had happened to my little girl?"

The next day she held the nurses in rapt attention. She had them gathered around the bed, striving for their total attention. "Listen to me," she commanded. "This is what you have to do." With that, she started a waving of the fingers of her right hand up the middle of her torso, over her face and her head, down the back of her neck, and when she couldn't reach anymore, she bent her arm in back and continued down her back, down to her foot and up her right leg. Intent on her instructions, she showed them again and again. "I'm trying to explain what's going on here," she said.

Oh, Alysa, Dave moaned inwardly, what *is* going on here? Besides seeing their daughter in such a horrendous state, the Conselyeas became increasingly frustrated as the doctors didn't seem to be doing anything. Other than draw blood, monitor blood pressure and check body temp, they had conducted no physical tests on Alysa to determine her illness. In their minds, it was all psychological.

"They even thought she was willfully creating the seizures so she could get drugs," Dave said, shaking his head. "They called them pseudo-seizures. If they were real seizures, we were told, she would have been incontinent."

Next, Alysa was given Haldol, a drug for schizophrenics to reduce anxiety. Within a couple hours she was completely listless and sedated. She became unaware of her surroundings. She would not eat. She wet the bed. Again, the doctors were talking about an MRI. Thus ended day three. Ken stayed the night.

Alysa became catatonic. She would communicate and then suddenly jerk rhythmically. Her eyes would burst open and shut, her tongue would stick out and every extremity would jerk. This did not stop! It continued for hours. Apparently, according to the doctors, she had a bad reaction to the drug. So, they cut the Haldol with Cogentin. Adding insult to injury, one doctor also said, "This happens sometimes to girls aged 18 to 21. It should all be over in about ten days."

"Hello! Are you an idiot?" Dave thought.

And then the clincher: she couldn't stay at that facility. All the doctors concurred that Alysa's problems were psychological. Bellville did have a psychiatric ward, but it was for patients who admitted themselves voluntarily. Alysa was incapable of admitting herself, and no one else was allowed to.

It all boiled down to money. Alysa had no health insurance. She was an adult so not covered by her parents' insurance. Therefore, she became a ward of the state. The doctors had mentioned the need for a spinal tap or an MRI, but they were never conducted.

Finally, exasperated, Dave pulled one of the residents aside. "How much does an MRI cost? I'll get the money. I'll pay for it somehow."

"Mr. Conselyea, money is not the issue here. We believe your daughter's problems are psychological."

Later, in the administrator's office, Dave took Linda's hand and turned to the hospital representative, "Could we get Alysa on Medicaid?"

"I'm afraid the paperwork would take too long to benefit her current situation," he said, discouragingly.

"You don't want her here because you're not sure you'll get your money?"

"I'm afraid we can do no more for your daughter at this facility. Could you please sign these forms consenting to her discharge?" Alysa was out.

An EMS ambulance arrived early that afternoon to transport Alysa, in her zombie-like state, to Pathways, in Pontiac, a medical clearinghouse that determines where indigent patients can be admitted for care. Linda rode in the ambulance with her daughter and Dave followed behind, alone.

"It was a blessing to leave Bellville. Supposedly, it's one of the best hospitals in the area, but not for Alysa," Linda recalled. "But here we were taking our daughter to Pathways, a place for street people and welfare recipients. We had prayed, where do we go? What do we do? We were going crazy. We had to trust that God would determine where Alysa was to go."

The physician at Pathways was quite sympathetic. After examining Alysa, he asked why a spinal tap had not been done?

Good question, Doc. Why hasn't anything been done? Dave thought to himself.

"Why don't you take her to Oakhill Memorial," he suggested. They have a psych ward and I'm sure they will admit her."

So, Alysa was cleared from Pathways and traveled by ambulance to Oakhill Memorial.

25

*　　*　　*　　*　　*

"Again, I rode with her in the ambulance," Linda recalled. "I was glad I was wearing my sunglasses because the tears were streaming down my face. 'Oh, Lord send me a miracle,' I prayed." Then Alysa, who hadn't spoken a word for two days opened up, "Hey, Mom! I just had a dream and I was at a big party."

"I'm thanking the Lord, and thinking, with all those drugs she's been given, I'll bet that was some party!" Suddenly, Alysa had another seizure.

"It was rush hour on I-75 when we started hurtling through traffic. The EMTs were tending to Alysa and like a dope I'm saying, 'Oh, this isn't a real seizure. This is a pseudo-seizure.' And they're looking at me and thinking, 'Right, lady, and we're Mickey Mouse and Goofy.'"

*　　*　　*　　*　　*

Alysa recovered from the seizure before arriving at Oakhill. Her blood pressure was elevated, her skin was blotchy red, and she had a fever. Nevertheless, Alysa was admitted and put in a room on a floor with all the loonies. It was a bitter pill to swallow. Worse, the Conselyeas were told that they could not stay.

"But we haven't left her side since she became ill," they protested, to no avail.

Devastated and distraught, they went home. Linda called her best friend, Cindy Schmidler, who had recently moved to Indianapolis, and asked first for prayer, and second, for Cindy to come and lend her moral support in person.

Interview with Linda Conselyea

The creamy, smooth complexion of this lovely, dark-haired woman belies the hardships Linda has faced. From her attitude and exuberance, one would never fathom the adversity she has borne. Marriage, divorce, single parenthood, cancer and fire had already scarred her life. But not her spirit.

In Linda's own words:

I have lived in rural Davisburg on Dixie Lake, twice: now, and as a child. My family moved to Ferndale, Michigan, when I was in the third grade. I graduated from Ferndale High School. I got

26

married soon out of high school in October of 1972 to an ordained minister I met at church. As a strong Christian, I never doubted that my husband would be a loving, compassionate mate. Unfortunately, his character and attributes were not biblical.

Shortly after Alysa was born August 30, 1974, we were scheduled to move to New Jersey where my husband had accepted a job. Faced with that move and the knowledge that the marriage was not working, I decided not to go. A minister that I greatly respected agreed with me that my mate was a "lousy husband." I was giving 125 per cent in the marriage, and he was giving zero. When I told my dad that I was going to file for divorce, he said, "What took you so long?"

I don't believe in divorce. I know that my divorce was a sin against God's plan for his people. Remorseful and sorry, I apologized to the Lord for not marrying who he intended for me to marry. On my knees I prayed that he could still use me for his kingdom. One of Satan's lies is that God will never use a sinful person for his purpose. I have learned otherwise. I do believe that Dave and I not having any children together was a result of my sin of divorce. But I accepted my barrenness and thanked God for Alysa.

I became a single mom with the usual difficulties and problems. We lived with my parents, off and on, from when Alysa was an infant until she was four years old. I had various jobs over a seven-year period to support Alysa and myself. In 1981, Ralph Conselyea hired me away from a secretarial job to work in his real estate office. He jokingly told me he hired me for his son. Dave and I worked side by side in the office for nearly two years and often double dated. Our first date with each other was in October of 1983.

My father knew from the first meeting that Dave was the one for me. Alysa, however, wasn't so easily won over. She hadn't shared me with anyone and she wasn't about to begin. The first time she accompanied us to dinner, she kept dropping her napkin under the table so she could look to see if we were holding hands. When I told her we planned to get married, she said, "No, you're not going to marry him. Tell him to leave. I'm gonna' go live with my gramma and that's how it's gonna be!"

We had a long talk that night. Her nine-year-old mind

absorbed everything I said and the next morning, she got up and called Dave to invite him over for breakfast. She had completely changed her mind. It didn't hurt that Dave lived in the house next door.

That Christmas Day, 1983, we were married. It just seemed the right thing to do. Dave had won tickets to the Super Bowl in Tampa, and that was our honeymoon. Dave and Alysa appeared before Judge Barry Grant, and his new daughter officially became Alysa Conselyea. We were all thrilled.

We had hoped to add to our family, but in October of 1985 some routine fertility tests discovered that I needed surgery on my fallopian tubes. With the holidays coming up, we decided to wait. The surgery was finally scheduled for May. The other surgery candidates and I watched a video on our procedures scheduled for the next day.

In the operating room when the doctors started what they thought was a normal tubal repair, they discovered suspicious tissue and expected cancer. Dave had left the waiting room to attend to a quick real estate matter nearby and had to be called back to talk to the physicians. They had consulted with an oncologist and all believed I had cancer. It was their preference that additional surgery, a hysterectomy, should be performed while I was still under anesthetic. That decision was so difficult for Dave to have to make on his own; but the doctors convinced him that waiting for the biopsy for a future surgery was life threatening. The result was a complete hysterectomy for me. We have both cried over that surgery, but the biopsy indeed turned out to be positive.

Afterwards, the doctors felt so bad that I found myself cheering them up. I knew I had to be strong or Dave and I both would fall apart. I relied on my faith. Everything had been in God's timing. It was a blessing. The ovarian and cervical cancers were of the silent nature. Had the surgery occurred earlier, the cancer may have gone unnoticed until too late. A year of chemotherapy followed, five days in a row each month. I was very sick, but I didn't lose my hair.

Our life was so good. Dave's work was stressful, and the hours were terrible, but he always treasured his time with Alysa and me. She became a loving and normal teenager. I was active in Bible Study Fellowship and other church endeavors. I chose to be a stay-at-home mom. I loved to make candy and pastries, and people were always begging for my specialty cakes and especially for my chocolate "cabbages."

In September of 1991, I opened my own shop, The Chocolate Cabbage Company, in the village of Clarkston. It offered chocolate cabbages, truffles, scones, pastries, cakes and high quality coffees and cappuccinos. It was unique. It took off right away. We had immediate success. The hours and hours of preparation of the goods were astounding. The shop was open from 8:00 a.m. to 10:00 p.m., six days a week. Preparing the items to sell during those 14 hours required another several hours before 8:00 a.m. plus continuous baking throughout the day. Sometimes I would even pull "all-nighters" just to meet customer demand.

I made so many new friends from running the shop. They would come in and sit down and we would visit. It was one of those friendly gatherings that probably saved my life. I was planning to work most of the night when some friends dropped in near closing. Dave came by, too, and he almost never came to the shop because he was afraid I'd find some work for him to do. So, we all talked and laughed until past 11:00 p.m. I kept wondering how I was going to get all of my Christmas orders done. Since I didn't get a good start that night, I decided to just go home and get a very early start in the morning. We got a phone call at 1:30 a.m. The shop was on fire! We drove back into the village and watched our sweet dreams go up in smoke.

The next day, as my dad was taking pictures of the remains, he came to me with tears in his eyes. My workroom was down the stairs beneath a trap door opening. That stairway had been completely destroyed by the fire.

"Linda, if you had been working, you would have been trapped," he told me with a catch in his voice.

I believe the Lord sent those friends into the shop that night to change my plans. They were a blessing!

The landlord was not a blessing. She had wanted to break my lease because another tenant was going to be more lucrative. She tried to blame the fire on us. Dave's building had a fire two months before, and she insinuated a connection between the two mishaps. We had money in the cash register, money in a drawer and money in a ceiling storage safe. Who burns up his own money? It was an ugly scene in all ways.

I know that "in all things God works for the good of those who love him, who have been called according to his purpose." I believe it was God who put me out of the candy and sweets business on December 4, 1992.

CHAPTER FOUR

Saturday, May 18
Day 6
We had to wait to see Alysa. No visitors allowed before 1:00
p.m. Finally got to see her. She looks like she is in a coma. John
and Cindy here from Indy. Had to leave at 3:00 p.m. sharp!
Second time we've had to leave her overnight. Still hasn't had
anything to eat or drink. I'm getting nervous about this.

Dave felt uneasy, to say the least. He couldn't observe the care
Alysa was getting and he hated her being alone. It was a joyless
night. Thank God for friends like Cindy and John. They had all
four prayed around Alysa's bedside. They prayed for healing and
for a better day tomorrow. The second prayer was answered.

Dr. Adam Baker had admitted Alysa to the psychiatric unit at
Oakhill Memorial, but he doubted that her condition was psychological. She had too many physical symptoms. He just hadn't
wanted to deny her a bed in the hospital. His misgivings plus the
medical opinions from other staff culminated in Alysa's being
moved to the sixth floor—a floor for physically ill patients.

The question of insurance had arisen again when Dave filled
out the admittance forms for Oakhill Memorial. He was instructed to contact Mary Jane Evans in Social Services to apply for
medical assistance.

He made the necessary call and reached Mrs. Evans' voice mail. He left his name and number. They played phone tag and eventually Dave explained their situation in a voice message. He received a letter regarding the application for Medicaid that required an immediate, ten-day response. Again, he called the number.

"You have reached the office of Mary Jane Evans. I will be out of the office for the next two weeks. Please leave a detailed message."

"This is Dave Conselyea. I'm just calling to let you know that I am responding immediately. I am sending in the application today, but I wanted to explain our situation to you as well."

He recounted Alysa's age, background and her emergency hospitalizations at Bellville and Oakhill Memorial. He described her incapacitation and her comatose state.

Alysa's Medicaid card arrived in the mail that very week. After only two or three phone calls, and one letter—and without any face-to-face meetings—the insurance problem was solved. It was so easy compared to all of the horror stories the Conselyeas had heard about getting on Medicaid.

"The Lord just took care of all of those details for us," Dave recalled. "It was incredible."

Dave and Linda arrived at Oakhill on the 19th and learned that Alysa was being transferred. They were overjoyed. At last they were going to find out what was wrong.

A senior resident in neurology, Dr. Dan Abraham entered their lives. A young Jewish man with caring eyes, he immediately showed compassion for the Conselyeas and their daughter.

"You may stay with your daughter as much as you want to," he told them. "A gynecological exam showed no evidence of trauma, although too much time has elapsed since she was in East Lansing for anything definitive. Your daughter is intact. On the other hand, the seizures your daughter has been having are very real and not psychotic."

Hallelujah! There was a physical reason! They were giddy with relief. Their excitement plummeted, however, when he continued.

"Alysa's EEG, the test that shows brain activity, reveals abnormal brain activity and multiple small seizures. We will try our best to determine the cause."

Dave immediately told the sympathetic doctor that Alysa hadn't had anything to eat or drink for five days.

"We'll get her on a feeding tube and give her liquids right away," he promised.

The long needed and crucial spinal tap, or lumbar puncture, was finally ordered. Linda and Dave spent the night with their child.

"The doctors at Oakhill Memorial were a godsend," recalled Linda. "The staff was wonderful—so conscientious and kind. They were truly an answer to prayer."

After the snow and ugly gray days of winter, springtime in Michigan was normally appreciated and enjoyed by the state's inhabitants. It could have rained nickels and bloomed dollar bills and the Conselyeas would not have noticed. Their singular focus was their daughter.

Tuesday, May 21
Day 9

5:15 a.m. Seizure. Dr. Raines, attending physician, in to see Alysa around 10:00. Dr. Abraham and Dr. Woods in at 11:00. Community Mental Health and State Attorney in and released psychiatric petition. I went to courthouse to file co-guardianship for Linda and me. Dr. Baker in to talk to Linda and Ken about the pet ferrets. 3:00 Doctors in to check on Alysa. She had a small seizure at 3:55 p.m. so they administered 1 mg Ativan. 4:05 They tried suctioning some secretions from Alysa's mouth. Spending the night. Lumbar puncture came back with high white blood cell count.

Alysa's court-appointed guardian had shown up at the hospital. "I'm here to sign a release of the psychiatric petition," he explained.

"You're what?" After a three-minute conversation, Dave was out the door and on his way to the courthouse to file co-guardianship papers for Linda and himself. Not to be in charge of his own daughter's care was more than he could bear.

Dr. Baker explained the meaning of high white blood cell counts to Linda and Ken.

"The normal CSF white blood cell count should be one. Alysa's count is 47. That means with that differential it is most likely a viral infection. We are going to classify it as viral encephalitis, or in layman's terms, a brain virus. It appears to be most similar to the herpes simplex virus, but we can't be sure. We need to discover what kind of virus it is and its origination. Ken, I understand that you and Alysa have a couple pet ferrets. We are trying to analyze anything that could have affected Alysa. We have tested for and ruled out Lyme disease, deer ticks and bovine contamination. Have your ferrets been sick? Could one of them have scratched or bitten Alysa?"

"No, I really don't think so," Ken said. "But if you need to do anything to them to find out what is wrong with Alysa, the ferrets are not important."

"No, no, I don't think we will even quarantine them. We just want to cover everything." With a slight sigh, the doctor added, "Unfortunately, herpes simplex can be an airborne virus, so we may never know how Alysa contracted it."

Wednesday, May 22
Day 10

1:50 a.m. Suctioned. Alysa had a seizure that lasted about 12 minutes. 4:15 a.m. Ativan 1 mg. Took about 10 minutes to work. 6:00 Gave Dilantin. Alysa choking. Nurse Alexis suctioned and that helped a lot. Respiratory in and started oxygen. Her pulse ox was 89%. 6:45 Attempted to suction again. 8:20 Dr. Canada (ophthalmology) checked her eyes per Dr. Baker. Drops will dilate eyes for up to 6 hrs. 9:00 Dr. Canada says Alysa's eyesight slightly fuzzy. 10:25 Seizure with mouth movement. Sat up for 25 minutes. Dave arrived hospital at 1:30 p.m. and they were finishing second EEG since we've been here. Dr. Canada back in and spoke briefly. Dr. Baker would like to do a skin culture from back of Alysa's neck. 7:00 Did another chest x-ray. Put air wraps on legs for circulation. 9:35 Sat up in bed for about 10 minutes. Eyes open. Gripping hands. Hazel, nurse, witnessed it. 10:15 Sat up. Lots of right arm movement. Eyes closed. Maybe seizure? 11:50 to 12:05 a.m. Alysa attempted to pull tubes off. Didn't let her sit up. Worked her legs until stimulators came off. 12:10 a.m. Temp. 99.9. 2:50 a.m. She woke up for about 5 minutes and sat up.

Alexis, Alysa's nurse, entered the room carrying an unusual-looking, light blue hose-like apparatus. She told the Conselyeas her intention.

"Dr. Abraham has ordered these air wraps for Alysa. We will put them on her legs to stimulate her circulation. Notice that the sequential segments are like a blood pressure cuff. They compress and release rhythmically and keep her blood moving."

"Are they uncomfortable?" Linda asked.

"Not at all; it's like a good massage."

"Gee, have you got one for the entire body? I'll volunteer to test it," Dave joked.

"We're working on it."

Later, even in her apparently comatose state, Alysa rubbed her legs continually and worked the Velcro loose. The air wraps flopped off her legs.

"It was hard to know if they hurt her or just bothered her. But once undone, the hissing of the air was quite annoying to us," Dave said. "She seemed distressed with the oxygen tube, too, and tried to pull it away from her face."

Thursday, May 23
Day 11

5:00 a.m. Woke up for 10 minutes. Linda rubbed back and she went back to sleep. 8:00 a.m. Seizure-like movements in eyebrows, hands, shoulders. Nurse Jane checked breathing and found it a little congested. 8:45 Dr. Stein, head of psychiatry, in to check Alysa. Chest x-ray at 9:10. Resting peacefully. Pastor Jim and church prayer warriors coming in to pray for her healing. 11:00 She sat up and gave hugs. Linda combed Alysa's hair. Stopped feeding for awhile and at 12:15 got Heparin shot (blood thinner) in stomach to help prevent clots. Drew 3 tubes of blood. 1:00 No fever. Sticking tongue out but not clenching or seizing. Dave called—he'll be up soon. When Dr. Abraham comes in, we will ask about feeding still being off. 2:00 Had bath and shampoo. 3:15 p.m. Nurse Ruby started food at 20cc per hour. Fever going down. She looks better today. Linda finally went home at 3:30. Alysa woke up at 5:00 p.m. and squeezed Linda Beaudoin's hands. Cindy S. called at 5:30 p.m. At 5:49 she sat up on her own, eyes wide open, reaching to pull tube away from her nose.

35

Fighting to sit up till 6:07. We put high top tennis shoes on her to help her feet from drooping. Nurse gave another tummy shot to help thin blood for legs. Put air wraps on legs again. 10:00 p.m. Linda came back.

Linda: "It was such a comfort to have Pastor Jim and others from the church pray for Alysa. They gathered around her bed; Jim took Alysa's hand and they asked God to protect and provide for Alysa in this time of trouble

Surprisingly, Alysa responded by giving hugs to everyone. I was touched. I walked down the hallway with Jim when they left and thanked him for coming."

She reentered Alysa's room just as an injection was being given in Alysa's stomach.

"Excuse me. Why is she getting a shot in her tummy? What is it for?"

"This is a shot of Heparin. It is needed to help prevent blood clots. When a patient like Alysa is in bed for long periods of time, there is always danger of a blood clot."

The aides entered to bathe Alysa. They had bundles of towels and blankets to place around her while they gave her a sponge bath.

"I'd like to help," Linda said. "Could I shampoo her hair?"

"Sure thing. Soon as we finish here. We'll just help lower the bed and move her up so you can get at her."

Linda filled the small pink basin with warm water. She stuffed towels all around Alysa's neck and over her throat. She carefully poured cups of water over Alysa's hair. Adding shampoo, she gently massaged Alysa's scalp.

"Alysa, Honey, I'll bet this feels so good. There's nothing like having nice, clean hair, is there? It always makes a woman feel so much better. I'm going to rinse now with clean water," she said as she ran the tap with warm water. She repeated pouring cups of water through Alysa's hair. Towels, Alysa and the floor received most of the water, but the task was completed. "Just a second. Then, we'll blow it dry."

Linda perfected the procedure over time as she and her mother tended to Alysa's personal care. It made her feel good to know that she was giving her some comfort.

That comfort was one of the few that Alysa had. The feeding tube was put back in that afternoon. It was a nasal gastric tube that entered her nose, went down her esophagus and into her stomach. Alysa didn't like it.

One of the nurses asked, "Was Alysa wearing sneakers when she was admitted?"

"As a matter of fact, she was."

"Are her street clothes still here—in the room?"

"Yes, they're in that bin over there. Do you want me to get them?"

"Yes, please. We want to keep stiffer shoes on her to keep her feet from drooping. We hope to prevent contractures, or shortening of the Achilles tendon. With shoes, she keeps her toes pointed upright. That helps," said the nurse as she finished tying the laces of the Nikes.

Lysa was all dressed up with no place to run.

Saturday, May 25
Day 13
3:15 a.m. Strong seizure lasting until 3:40. Temp=100.4. Right arm was hanging over side of bed then started flailing up and down. Alysa has not had bowel movement since May 13. Given suppository.

Sunday, May 26
Day 14
Suppository worked. And worked. And worked. Arms swollen. Stomach bloated. Nurse Janet thinks maybe liver dysfunction because ammonia and enzymes are up. Dr. Corbin said she is less responsive. Moving her mouth as if to talk (no sound) for about five minutes.

The functioning of the human body is a miracle in itself. Doctors, nurses and family regard the normal functioning of a patient's body as a positive sign. One of the good signs is the natural elimination of waste. Consequently, the Conselyeas recorded the frequency and the nature of Alysa's bowel movements in the daily journal.

Suffice it to say that with the nurses' busy schedules, they were usually not the ones to keep Alysa clean. That task fell to whoever was at her bedside: Linda, Dave, Sylvia, Ken, and Ken's mom. "It was just something we did," Ken would recall later.

Monday, May 27
Day 15
Dr. Baker says some pneumonia in left lung. Will have to change antibiotics. He thinks it's a good idea to put feeding tube in stomach due to sinus complication. Nurse called Dr. Corbin to look at her because of mouth movements and pulse rate high. New drug given to fight virus found in urine, Ticarcillin.

"I think we'll discontinue the NGT—feeding tube—and replace it with a gastrostomy," Dr. Raines told Linda. "Alysa is having sinus complications with the nasal tube."

"Exactly what is a gastrostomy, Doctor?"

"It doesn't require an incision. It's just like a poke into her stomach with a tiny tube. She will be much more comfortable, and believe me, she'll like it better than the nose tube."

So one tube and wire was exchanged for another. Progress.

Friday, May 31
Day 19
2:15 a.m. Linda cleaned Alysa up after bowel movement. 4:45 a.m. Got pain shot so she can rest. Temp, pulse and BP all normal. 6:50 More blood drawn. Linda, Linda B., Grandma Rivers, Denise Moffett, and Carrie Komisarz gave Alysa bath and shampoo. 2:00 p.m. Had EEG. 5:00 p.m. Temp= 97. B.P.= 117/70. 8:05 Temp= 97.4. Between 9:30 and 10:00 Alysa tried to cough and was not able to. Nurse Sally walked into room and nurse Karen suctioned Alysa orally with a suction catheter. Sally got pulse. Oxygen readings were down to 63% (dangerously low) for her blood oxygen. Color poor. Respiration extremely labored. Alysa fought suctioning by biting through catheter. Put her on 100% oxygen. NRB (non re-breather mask), and SaO2 going up to 85% with more suctioning. They bagged her and were having difficulty. Dr. stated Alysa had hipoxic and acidotic levels of blood gas. Color still poor. Doctors and nurses running in and out. Lots of equipment brought in to revive her. Decided to intubate her to get

necessary oxygen to lungs and brain. Alysa needed 4mg Ativan and fought intubation. After intubation, oxygen level back up to 99-100%. Heart rate regular. Chest x-ray ordered. Alysa transferred to ICU. A very close call. We almost lost her.

CHAPTER FIVE

Linda and Dave reacted to Alysa's new emergency with growing anxiety and concern. Her hospital bed was placed in a curtained area with three other patients in the ICU. Nurses and doctors swarmed around her attending to her needs. Finally, Dr. Abraham took them aside.

"I know you are worried about all that is happening to Alysa right now. I just want you to know that this is a minor setback. The emergency has been averted and her vital signs are stable. She will receive constant monitoring here. This is a good place for her to be. I would suggest that you go home and get some rest." He looked at his chart in his hands then fixed his eyes on Linda's. "Don't worry about your daughter."

It was 1:00 a.m. when Linda finally went home. Ken and Dave went to the hospital beds that had been assigned to them.

Dave: "Once the staff realized that we were not ever going to leave Alysa, I think they took pity on us. We camped out in the lounge until they offered us an alternative. The room was on the sixth floor and was very spacious by hospital standards. It had two beds with individual TV's and an adjoining bathroom.

"Ken and I would take turns during the night to check on Alysa. We were always readily available for consultations. It was truly a blessing."

Ken's mom—referred to as Linda Two, in order to differentiate between Linda Conselyea and her—arrived early that morning after the guys had left for work to maintain the continuous 24-hour vigil. On her watch, a Dr. Anne Bradford examined Alysa.

"We think it would benefit Alysa if we give her a central line in her neck. That way she is more readily accessible for intravenous drug administration," she announced.

"Have you done this procedure before?" Linda Two bluntly asked.

Obviously not expecting to be challenged, the doctor tilted her head, "I beg your pardon?"

"I'm sorry, I didn't mean to seem impertinent. You see, I had a botched central line when I had surgery and it has given me trouble ever since," she explained.

"I can assure you that I have performed many of these procedures—all without incident."

So it was a shock when Linda walked in to see her daughter that afternoon. The respiratory tube poked its way from her throat and out her mouth, the feeding tube invaded her stomach, and the central line protruded from her neck. And still she had no idea what was happening to Alysa.

Linda: "I was emotionally and physically drained, but always when something seemed really bad, something good would happen. That day two young women from the Bardha Salon came to visit Alysa. They brought food and goodies for us, and the front desk receptionist sent her loose cash and told us to have dinner—her compliments. People were phenomenally good to us."

The next day, Sunday, Linda again experienced opposite feelings. At church, Linda physically leaned on Dave and he supported the weight of their shared burden, their sick daughter. During the service, Pastor Jim told of Alysa's plight and then questioned his congregation in the packed auditorium.

"How many of you are willing to commit to pray for Alysa for one hour every day?"

The Conselyeas were awestruck by the response.

Dave: "Almost every hand in the room was raised. Linda and I could not hold back our tears. We looked around and saw people who didn't even know us, or Alysa, volunteering to pray for our precious daughter. God is so good!"

Monday, June 3
Day 22

9:00-11:30 a.m. Dave here with Alysa. Blood test. Suctioned 2-3 times. A little anxious with all the doctors seeing her today. Hopefully taking ventilator off tonight or tomorrow. Linda and Sylvia here by 10:30. Dave back at 3:00. Pastor Jim and Carol here to check on Alysa. Removed tube protector and hope she won't try to bite through it. Doing an ultrasound on her legs to see if there are blood clots. Alysa may have had a seizure tonight. They gave her Dilantin and Ativan.

The roller coaster continued on Monday. The doctors hoped to wean Alysa off the ventilator. They had worried about potential brain damage due to lack of oxygen from Friday's episode, but all the reports showed no threat. The Conselyeas learned that a patient became more dependent on the ventilator the longer she was connected. The ventilator, or respirator, breathed for the patient if she did not initiate the breaths herself.

Pneumonia and mucous plugs were a constant threat to the patient, making suctioning out the mucous or phlegm an ongoing procedure. Weaning transpired when the machine could be shut off for incremental periods of time: a few minutes at first then gradual increases of time.

Dave kept himself pumped up by staying connected with his strength, his God. "I am believing God for a total, 100% recovery," he wrote in the journal.

Linda: "It was so hard to be a mom and look at your daughter. With all those tubes plus the bite block to prevent her from clamping her teeth on the tube—she looked so pathetic. Her lips were three times their normal size. Blisters erupted and infection followed. The nurses would scrape her lips and clean them. Sometimes, I would just have to avert my eyes. It was one of those moments when Dr. Abraham came into the room."

"Hi, Linda. How's it going today?"

"I guess all right. Poor Alysa looks so pitiful. And I always wonder if she is in any pain."

"I don't know if this will be of any comfort to you, but I've brought this book for you. My aunt read it after my uncle died, and I just thought it might help."

42

He handed her a copy of Rabbi Harold Kushner's *When Bad Things Happen To Good People*. The tenderhearted Dr. Abraham was reaching out to the hurting parents, and his kind act brought pure joy. But Linda later said that the theology of the book was contrary to her beliefs. Kushner apparently believes that God has limited control and is even outraged by the unfairness on earth and has no power to change chaotic events.

Linda never questioned the power of her God.

A double whammy hit the next day. After a meeting with Dr. Beltz, the ICU pulmonologist, and Jill, his assistant, a decision was reached to perform a tracheostomy on Alysa. Sylvia was with Linda and they discussed it. Then Linda called Dave.

"Dave, the doctors have suggested another procedure for Alysa. They want to give her a tracheostomy."

"What's that? I've heard of someone being 'trached,' but I guess I never knew why."

"Well, it sounds better for Alysa. She wouldn't have the tube down her throat. They say she'd be more comfortable and that it's easier on her. She's been on the respirator for more than a week, so they think it's time to do the trache. It's a surgical opening in the front of her neck to pass the tubes into her lungs. So what do you think?"

"My main concern is Alysa. If this is easier for her, then I'm all for it. I'll be over there in a couple hours. Give Lysa my love."

"Okay, I will."

Linda replaced the receiver and reentered Alysa's area. A nurse gently tucked the bedclothes around Alysa and reached for her wrist to take her pulse. The train of nurses, aides and doctors chugged unceasingly in the ICU. The parade of visitors almost equaled the professional staff. Mike and Lisa McCulloch, their friends and attorney, tapped on the wall.

"Hello, can we come in?" he asked. Bundled in his arms he held a dozen beautiful red roses.

"Oh, Mike. Lisa. How nice of you to come. And look at those roses. Alysa, see what Mike and Lisa brought you," Linda said, guiding Mike closer to Alysa's bed.

"Hi there, sport. We just wanted to see how you were doing."

He turned to Linda. "How is she doing?"

"She's stable at the moment. They have scheduled a tracheostomy on the 5th. She won't have that tube down her trachea after the procedure. I'm hoping that will make her more comfortable. We are just taking one day at a time and asking God to help us through it."

After they left, Linda found a place to temporarily display the roses. Flowers weren't allowed in the ICU and there wasn't any room among the equipment that was keeping her daughter alive. She vowed to keep all of Alysa's flowers—to dry them—and later Alysa would know how much everyone cared.

The tracheostomy was performed on the 6th—on time by hospital standards. It went well and the Conselyeas praised God for that. It may have been good for Alysa, but it was another foreign protuberance that was difficult to view. The nurses tended to it proficiently and with care. The trache itself was inserted through an incision, or ostomy, in the throat and the tubes went into Alysa's lungs. There was a strap around Alysa's neck to hold it on. The ventilator connected to a hole in the trache. A curved tube or cannula was removed and changed a couple times each day. The area was kept sterile at all times and sterile gloves were mandatory. Preventing foreign matter from entering the lungs was primary.

Friends and visitors were heavenly gifts. Andrea Denyes, a former cheerleader from high school, entered Alysa's room with trepidation. She didn't know where to look or to whom to speak. Alysa had her eyes open, but was non-responsive.

"Hi, Alysa. How ya' doin?" She asked. She then turned to Linda. "Mrs. Conselyea, can she hear me or see me?"

"We aren't sure, Andrea. But we still speak to her and tell her things. She may understand more than we think she can. Why don't you talk to her for awhile?"

Andrea approached the bed, took a gulp of breath and launched into a monologue.

"Alysa, do you remember when we won the cheerleading competition during our senior year? It was such a thrill. I can remember your reaction. Of course we were all screaming and crying and jumping around, but you were so excited you started doing flips on the gym floor. You were amazing when you did the flips. You were the most limber one on the cheerleading team and no one could do them as well as you.

"I remember the party at your house, too, when we t.p.'d old

44

Mr. Fartface. Oh, sorry," she said, turning to Linda and grimacing at her gaff.

"That's okay. I think the name fits him well, from what I heard," Linda said, putting Andrea at ease.

"Anyway, that was the most fun. When he caught you, I thought you were a goner. We had some great times, didn't we?" She paused. "Well, I just thought I'd come in and say hi. I hope you are better soon."

"Thanks for coming by, Andrea. It's nice to know her friends think about her."

"I do hope she is better soon. Will she be?"

"We're counting on it."

Laurie Hall and Pat Toth were Linda's prayer partners. She would share with one or both of them on a daily basis and they would pray for Alysa and for her family. They were only a part of the support team of over 330 known people who endured throughout. Linda's sister, Carol, came to the hospital daily. John and Cindy Schmidler called often, sent cards and gifts. They knew that Alysa collected classic Winnie the Pooh items. A gift had arrived for Alysa. Linda took it to Alysa's bedside.

"John and Cindy sent you a present. Do you want to open it?" Linda asked, knowing that Alysa wouldn't respond and that she was not able to even hold the gift.

"I'm going to help you take the ribbon and the paper off. Let's see. What is it? Oh, Alysa! It's a music box. A Pooh music box. Isn't that adorable? Let's listen and hear what tune it plays."

Linda wound the key and held the box up to Alysa's ear.

"It's the Winnie the Pooh theme song, Alysa. Can you hear it?"

Later, she wedged the music box between the wall and the bright yellow boom box sitting on the windowsill.

Friday, June 7
Day 26

8:20 p.m. Going down to see Alysa. She had lumbar puncture sometime between 6:00 and 8:00. MRI at 8:30. Lasted an hour. She was very still—had to be sedated. MRI shows small lesion this time. Doctors not recommending brain biopsy. Consulting doctor from Bellville, Dr. Bubala, to discuss this with us. Other than

Dilantin, no other drugs today. Ken staying the night as usual. Dave going to Rivers to be with Linda for the first time in weeks.

Alysa had to be sedated for the MRI. Otherwise, her constant robotic movements would make an MRI impossible. One must remain absolutely still for the imaging to be read. Alysa constantly moved her body in jerky, robotic, stiff gestures. Her hands, fingers, head and shoulders worked in sync like a white-faced mime on a San Francisco street corner. The doctors did not know if her movements were caused by the virus, the seizures or from the drugs she was given—one of several unknowns.

Dave: "We didn't know if we should be happy or sad over the results of the MRI. It appeared to be good news that there was something in the brain—something that could be causing all of her symptoms. Yet, a lesion was another mystery to us. A renowned neurosurgeon was brought in to consult. Ken, Linda, Linda Two and I all discussed the findings with Dr. Abraham and Dr. Baker."

"Dr. Bubala is willing to get a biopsy from Alysa's brain. It would mean drilling a hole through her skull and into her brain to take a tiny bit of the lesion for testing," Dr. Baker said. "I am not totally convinced that there would be enough yield to determine the cause of the virus. The decision is yours to make."

"Doctor, what would you do if it were your own child?" Linda asked.

"I would not have it done," the infectious disease specialist responded.

"It could be construed that we did not do everything possible to discover the origin of your daughter's illness," cautioned Dr. Abraham.

"You mean, that the doctors are afraid of a malpractice lawsuit if this test is not done, is that it?" Dave asked.

Dr. Abraham didn't bridle at the question. "We all want to know what is making Alysa so ill, but I agree with Dr. Baker. The chances of getting what we need from the biopsy are slim to none at this time."

"I am willing to sign an affidavit that we won't sue if this test is not performed," said Linda.

Nodding his head in agreement, Dave said, "Since it's a long

46

shot, I don't want it done either. We won't file a malpractice suit."

Ken, as usual, was always pleased when he was included in the process of the Conselyeas' decision-making. He didn't feel that he should give his opinion on the brain biopsy, but he was relieved when the idea was rejected.

*   *   *   *   *

On Sunday, June 9, Dave told Linda he had a surprise for her. He drove toward their home in Davisburg.

"Where are we going? Are we going home?" Linda asked. She hadn't stepped foot into their home since Sunday, May 12.

"Yep, I've got something to show you." The lake sparkled on this beautiful early summer day. Dave parked the car in the driveway, opened the car door for Linda and grabbed her hand. He partly tugged her into the breezeway that was their entry and said, "Close your eyes."

"Dave, what is it?"

He led her through the kitchen and stopped short of what before had been the dining room. "Okay, open!" he said.

"You did it! I can't believe it. How nice of you to arrange for it—especially with all that has been going on. Dave, I thank you. I really do," Linda said, giving her generous husband a hug and kiss.

Somehow, Dave had found time to purchase the furniture that the two of them had seen in a builder friend's model home open house. The peach-colored sectional sofa and matching plaid chair were all shoved into the compact living room and there was no room to walk between the pieces. But still, it was lovely. Dave had a few things to tend to, so Linda wandered outside to the dock.

Linda: "It was very difficult for me to be in the house. I couldn't bear to walk into Alysa's room and see her things. I sat on the dock with my knees pulled up to my chest, my arms wrapped around them, and started to cry. My sunglasses partly shielded my grief had any neighbors been watching. I hoped no one would come talk to me. I felt as empty as Alysa's room."

Interview with Dave Conselyea

Dave Conselyea is captivating. Genuine and happy, he displays a stereotypical salesman's personality. His photo can be found in the dictionary under "nice guy." That photo would be with a ponytail if it were AAI, After Alysa's Illness, or it would be with clean-cut, short hair if it were BAI, Before Alysa's Illness.

In Dave's words:

I date everything in my life as either "before" or "after" Alysa got sick. It has been, by far, the most all-consuming event in my life. My entire focus has changed. The only thing that is important to me is my family. Time with my family is a gift from God. God has always been in my life.

I was known as "Preacher Boy" when I was in middle school and high school. I carried my Bible with me everywhere, and most of my speeches in speech class were sermons. In today's environment, a kid like me wouldn't have a chance. I started Bible studies in school and was always talking to my friends…yes, I did have friends…about being saved. I was saved when I was eight years old. Even as a young child, when asked what I wanted to be when I grew up, my pat response was "a minister, a missionary, an evangelist, or a Realtor like my dad."

I attended Bob Jones University in Greenville, South Carolina, and hated it! It was so restrictive; it was unbelievable. You could get demerits just for walking off campus. I failed miserably and left after one year. I came home and went to Detroit Bible College, which is now William Tyndale. It is a liberal arts school with a Christian emphasis.

I married an 18-year-old girl when I was almost 21. The marriage lasted three-and-one-half years from start to finish. Of all the people in my family to get a divorce, it's hard to believe I was the one. I believe the scriptures teach against divorce. My wife was what we call a "completed Jew." Born to Jewish parents, she and her family professed knowing Christ. It was an amicable parting. She wanted to go to California and I wanted to stay. Before we parted ways, she told me I was one of the nicest guys she ever knew. I paid for the divorce; we split everything 50/50 and my dad even gave her a car when she left.

I did carry some guilt for breaking the marriage vow that I made with the Lord. Truly remorseful, I admitted my wrongdoing to God. It was a youthful mistake. But like the prodigal son, I believe God forgave me and gave me a clean slate. I don't believe that the sins of the fathers visit the children unless they are sins of ongoing disobedience. That God allowed me the love of my life in Linda is proof of his wanting only good for me. It's uncanny that both Linda's and my marriage of our youth dissolved partly because of geography. I guess our roots are solidly planted in the metro Detroit area.

I had the will, the background and the training for three of my childhood vocational choices, but I decided to test the fourth. I took the real estate course without telling my dad, and I passed with flying colors. I joined my dad's firm, Ralph Conselyea, Realtor. That was after all of the national franchises, like Century 21, had entered the field and dad was down to 12 or 15 agents. In his heyday, he had 25-35 people in his organization. We were located in downtown Royal Oak.

I am the youngest of four children. My two brothers and sister never had any interest in real estate, so with great enthusiasm my father welcomed me into the firm. When I started working for my dad, I was in my rebellion days, or at least that's what I call them. I was twenty-five, divorced and enjoying myself. Still, the Lord tugged on me, and I knew when I was in the will of the Lord and when I wasn't. I was dating several women when I first asked Linda out. In fact, Linda was working at the office and she answered the phone when all of my girlfriends would call.

I asked Linda's deadbeat boyfriend of two years if I could take her out to hear Smokey Robinson. Linda was dating a chef who never took her anywhere, and he granted his permission. As soon as we went out that night, I knew I was going to marry this woman.

I tactfully untangled all of my other relationships so I could concentrate on Linda. I was smitten. Two-and-one-half months later, we were married. It's been basically wedded bliss ever since. Linda is just the greatest thing in my life.

I knew Alysa since she was seven or seven-and-a-half. I rented Linda a house that was next door to mine. Alysa was used to seeing me, but she expected her mom to marry the chef.

In recent years, people are confused when I am out with Alysa. I am 18 years older than she is, but I have retained my boyish good looks. Seriously, some give me disapproving looks. Daughter? Wife? Wife's sister? People I have mild acquaintance with might comment, "Boy, you must have been married pretty young" or "How old are you?" I never let it bother me. I hate the term step-daughter, so I always say she's my daughter.

My lifelong philosophy has always been that God is in control. I have never felt hate for anyone and I have never blamed anyone for anything. I am just so grateful that God chooses to bless me. During Alysa's illness, I felt terrible for Alysa and was more worried for Linda, her mother. My constant prayer was "Lord, you've got to work something out here." All along, I felt that the Lord was going to heal her; I clung to Romans 8:28, "And we know that in all things God works for the good of those who love him, who have been called according to his purpose." I knew he was going to touch her life.

Just because God is in control doesn't mean that I always did the right thing. Even though I trusted the Lord, I still crumbled under the pressure of my business. In 1986, I created a partnership with another man in industrial and commercial real estate. The stress of this new business, with my dad and my wife all in one office, became too much. I'm not proud to admit it, but I just took off. I was gone for about 10 days. I just started driving across the country. About the seventh day, I finally had the decency to call home. Linda met me in California and we talked things out on the drive back to Michigan. Changes were made. We dissolved the partnership, I started a satellite office located on Crooks Road, and Linda became an 'at home' mom.

That is my office today. Now my dad comes in and does a little work there. He will never retire. He loves the business too much. He and mom have lived in 20 different homes. Fifteen out of the 20 he brokered through his business. The only problem is the pinball machine. Their current home is smaller than all of their previous residences, so he moved his pinball machine into my office and comes in to play. It drives me crazy! I ask him if he can leave it alone for awhile and he says he is just about to get his best score! It is a trifle distracting.

My true retreat is our home on Dixie Lake. When I saw that property, I fell in love with it. The house was owned by a retired widower, so you can imagine its limitations. But seeing the water every day is worth the small space. I acted somewhat impulsively and didn't pray about it before making the decision to purchase it. But Linda said "okay" and we bought it! I love the privacy this retreat allows us.

That dream property stayed vacant from May 12 to December 12, 1996, because during that time we lived at Linda's parents, the Rivers. Linda was back only twice: once in June to see new furniture and again in October to get some clothes. It was a hard time.

Interview with Ralph Conselyea

Dressed in his pinstriped business suit, 83-year-old Ralph Conselyea still arrives at the office every weekday morning at 8:00 o'clock. His work is his haven for collecting friendships old and new—his office a showcase for memories of a lifetime of caring about people. Signed photos of two of the five presidents he personally met grace the wall along with aerial pictures of the Royal Oak commercial properties that catapulted his real estate success. Regaled tales of years long gone intermixed with current situations jump the agile hurdles of his mind. But Alysa's illness brings him up short. With a lump in his throat and tears at the ready, he speaks with the emotion known only by another grandparent. "She's my granddaughter!"

Ralph shares his life stories:

Our origins are from France. The first Conselyeas came to Michigan in 1817. My grandmother was a Christian Scientist, but my mother and our family were Presbyterians. After my father died when I was eleven, we went to church with my grandmother. All the women in my life—my grandmother, mother and my sisters—were members of the WCTU or Women's Christian Temperance Union. I guess they convinced me because I've never touched a drop of beer, liquor or wine in all my years.

When I met Roselind, she lived in St. Clair, Michigan, and I lived up the road in Port Huron where I was a shoe salesman at Sperry's. I got a job with Detroit Edison as a meter reader and that's what I was doing when we started dating. Judge Black, a fellow St. Clair judge hired by Roselind's father, asked me to serve as the conservator of her dad's estate after he died. The judge knew my dad from the Spanish American War. I was twenty-one and Roselind was twenty. The judge asked how long we'd been dating and I told him two years. He asked why didn't we just get married? So we did. Maybe the paperwork was easier than arranging a conservator. It was kind of crazy. Being foolish, we tore down the family home and built a new one designed by the

51

architect Walter Whythe.

I had always wanted to run a men's wear store and we opened one in St. Clair. It did very well. I joined the Lions Club and have belonged to it for 60 years. We decided we wanted to open another store and we came down and ate at Hedges, the big restaurant at 10 Mile and Woodward. And to our good fortune, right near it was a men's store that had gone out of business. That was our second store on Main Street. At the same time I bought out a distressed store in Coldwater for the fixtures and the stock. We then sold our stores and a buyer came to us for the new house we built, so we moved to Royal Oak.

Next, the war came. I got a job at N.A. Woodworth's as an inspector on the line. By then, I knew all the storeowners in town so when the plant had a shortage of cheesecloth that was desperately needed to wrap the valves, I knew where to get it. I saved the day, or night as it was the night shift, and word got out. I was just 25 and I got hired as a manager of 7,000 people for Graham Page Motors. The management had me deferred because they said I was vital to the plant and the war effort. After the war, I wanted to work in men's wear again, but there were no vacant stores to buy. I saw an ad in the newspaper for a manager of a shoe store. I knew I could do that, so I had an interview with the owner at his Royal Oak store. He needed a manager for his Hamtramak store. I told him I wanted Royal Oak. A woman shopper helped make the decision.

She was leaving the store without any purchases. I couldn't help myself. I asked her if she had found what she wanted and she said no. I proceeded to discover just what exactly she wanted and I helped her to get it. Nice shoes were about a dollar in those days. When I was finished, she happily departed with seventeen dollars worth of shoes, handbags and stockings. The owner had watched me and said I could manage the Royal Oak store and he'd send that manager over to Hamtramak.

I joined the Board of the Salvation Army in 1940 and am still on the Board today. I built a network of people in the community through the Lions, the morning coffee klatches and other connections. If you're nice to people and like them, it pays off.

My store became the cash-checking location for the operators at Bell Telephone. Those gals would come in to cash their checks and buy shoes, too. In fact, many of them bought shoes for their relatives in Canada where shoes weren't available. They'd scuff the soles and send them across the border. We sold nearly 32 pairs a week just to them. Once I made a bad mistake. I ordered 1,000 pair of women's boots with the fur cuff when I should have only ordered about 200. We had a big snowstorm and women were lined up out to the corner to get boots. Other stores were calling to see if I could send them some. We sold every pair. The company gave me a $500 bonus for my "mistake." They wanted to move me to the Detroit store, and I didn't want to go. So I took a leave of absence and that's when Paul Morrison talked me into real estate. That's what I've been doing ever since.

I began by selling homes and properties for 17 different builders. I built some $30,000 homes on some city property I bought and today they go for $185,000. I had nine guys working for me in those days. Only three of them are alive today. We always made sure that the homes were sold right—that the people were taken care of. The commercial buildings accounted for the firm's foundation, but I always liked the residential part of the business best. David surprised me with his real estate license and he came into the business about 18 years ago.

Roselind and I have four children: Karen, Bill, Fred and Dave. Karen was in college when Dave was born. We lived in 20 different houses while the kids were growing up. Roselind liked the change and she loved working in the yards. That's always been her passion. She's been kind of forgetful recently—doesn't quite remember things. We have 16 grandkids.

We've always been close to Alysa because she's the one who lived nearby. We've seen her more often than the others who live away. So, when she got sick, we were really knocked over by it. I had never had anything that serious in my whole life. Roselind and I would go to the hospital and just stand and look at her for 15 to 30 minutes. She would be absolutely motionless. We'd go day after day and there would be no change. Then when she did open her eyes, she would just stare. It was so hard to bear. But it was really hard on Roselind. We had to stop going because it upset her so much. Linda doesn't know it but I went by myself many times. I don't think anyone realized just how deeply we felt.

I have a deep faith in God and in Christ. I've never felt like I had to do things that would outwardly show my faith. My faith is inward. I've shown my love by how I've treated people and how I've lived my life. I'm a Protestant but I've gone to so many different churches, I'm not a stickler for denominations. Besides the Christian Scientist and the Presbyterians, I've been a Methodist and a Baptist and almost a Lutheran. There's not just one church; there are many. And I have no quarrel with any of them—except atheists. And they're really missing the truth.

CHAPTER SIX

Many medical procedures were presented, considered and performed over the next several days. Determining the cause of Alysa's illness was a priority. A transesophogeal echocardiogram, or TEE, was done. A scope was inserted down her throat and placed behind her heart to see if tissue or blood had broken off and gone to the brain to cause a stroke. The results were negative. Alysa had a very strong heart.

A liver scan was performed as well as an ultrasound for blood clots. No definitive results. A Groshong catheter was introduced to replace the central IV line. Now there would be a more permanent port, or avenue, for medication and blood drawing; it would be longer lasting than the central IV that had to be changed every other week.

Alysa contracted a blood bacteria; stronger antibiotics were administered to fight the bacteria. Dave and Linda wrote into their journal unfamiliar medical terms and hard to spell and pronounce drugs.

Linda said, "It was the beginning of our lay person MD degree."

All the time that Alysa was in intensive care, she was nonresponsive but continually moving. Dave: "For lack of a better term, we called it a catatonic state. People thought we were being hopeful when we read and talked to Alysa. We did have hope—

and faith in God. I remember telling her at about that time, 'Lys, I'm in bad need of a haircut, but there's no time. You've got to get well so I won't look like a shaggy dog.'"

"These movements could be caused by several factors," one doctor explained to Dave and Linda. "It could be a seizure. They could be drug-related or be side effects from drugs, especially the Haldol that she received when she was first hospitalized. Unfortunately, her neurological symptoms could be masked by the drugs."

Linda and Dave became the best judges of Alysa's agitation and reaction to certain drugs. In fact, Linda discovered what elevated Alysa's fevers. Dilantin was the culprit. The doctors didn't see her on a 24-hour basis, and each new doctor was always shocked to witness her constant movements.

Linda: "Dr. Raines, Alysa's attending physician seemed to react daily according to Alysa's progress. Very dapper in his spats and stylish gray hair, his feelings registered on his face. If things were good, he was happy. If things were bad, he was down. He treated her as if she could respond. We loved him!"

"How's my girl, today?" Dr. Raines would ask, taking hold of Alysa's limp hand. "You look good to me. Your color is good. Is everyone treating you well? You know, my youngest daughter is a little older than you. I'll bet you two would be good friends. She's in school out east. I sure do miss her. Well, you keep everyone in line around here, okay?" he would say as he placed a kiss on her forehead.

Many of the doctors were kind-hearted and caring. When told that Alysa had suffered from cysts on her ovaries, Dr. Woods sympathized. She told Linda, "I think I'll have an ob-gyn test run. Alysa looks uncomfortable to me and maybe she is having pain from the cysts. She has enough problems. If we can eliminate any of her distress, we should."

Physical therapy and occupational therapy occurred daily. The therapist would move Alysa's hands and arms and massage and move her feet. Otherwise, the muscles would become atrophied, or wasted. "It's good for circulation, too," one therapist explained. "And it can keep her from getting pneumonia."

Occupational therapy has a wide range of interpretation. One thinks of training for a job, or some sort of skill. For Alysa at this time of her illness, it meant getting up and sitting in a chair. This was no easy feat with all the wires and tubes coming out all over her body. Yet, it was exhilarating to the family to have Alysa do something so normal as sitting in a chair. Moments away from the hospital bed were hopeful moments.

Dr. Renee Thomas, a tall, dark-haired woman in her late 40's, had been at a party when she heard about Alysa's case. She waltzed into Alysa's room at midnight after leaving the party.

"Hi, I'm Dr. Thomas. I'm an ob-gyn and I'd like to help Alysa if I can," she said, introducing herself to Dave.

"I'm Dave Conselyea. It's very good to meet you. We don't get many doctors or visitors this time of night."

"I was at a party and some of the staff were there and they were discussing your daughter. I wanted to come and help. I'd like to examine her and then discuss possible remedies, if that is all right with you?"

"Of course it is. Do you mean right now?"

"Sure. No time like the present."

"I was just about to get some more coffee. I'll step out and you can examine Alysa."

The doctor approached Alysa. "Hi, Honey. I'm Dr. Thomas and I'm going to give you a simplified pelvic exam, okay? I'll be very gentle and it will only take a couple minutes." She conducted the exam and was finished when Dave returned.

"What I'd like to recommend is to give Alysa a shot of Deproprevera. It would prevent menstrual cycles for three months. It has no long-term effect on fertility. It would relieve her of the bother of periods. Also, I think the injection will eliminate the pain from the ovarian cysts."

Dave, always a "naturalist" with matters of reproductive interference, relented, "We just want our daughter to be made as comfortable as possible. Your suggestion is fine with me if it will help solve even one little problem. Doctor, I appreciate your help."

"By the way, does she always have these arm motions?"

"Yes. Sometimes it's even worse. This is a calm period for Alysa."

"I don't think I've ever seen anything quite like it. It's somewhat disconcerting, isn't it?"

"Yes, it really is. It's funny, though. She's been doing this for

57

a month, and it's crushing to admit that we're getting used to it. We're still in total disbelief of the entire illness and all of its ramifications," Dave said, slowly shaking his head.

"I can understand how you feel. Well, I'd better be off. I've got early rounds tomorrow. And I never know when one of my patients might start labor. It was a pleasure to meet you."

"Same here," Dave said as he slid open the curtain for her.

The next day, the speech therapist introduced herself to Linda Two.

"Alysa isn't speaking," Linda Two said. "So, exactly what do you do for her?"

"We just want to stimulate her mouth and her tongue. I'll rub this lip gloss on her lips, sort of a massage, and rub her tongue with this sponge," she explained.

Linda Two watched, and asked, "Now, what is that?"

Using a Q-tip-like object, the therapist said, "This is a flavored instrument. By rubbing it on the patient's gums and tongue, it stimulates the taste buds and massages the gums."

As the therapist gently parted Alysa's lips and moved the Q-tip around, Alysa had no reaction or response to the exercise; but it was fascinating to Linda Two.

"Boy, you learn something new every day around here. I would never have thought that was part of speech therapy," she said.

Not surprisingly, Alysa was allergic to many of the drugs she was given. Amphotericin, Vancomycin, Haldol, Dilantin and all sulfa drugs were problematic. She also developed a terrible rash from the tape that was used to keep lines, tubes and wires in place. Blisters appeared first and then the site would become infected. Above her bed a large sign read, "Paper Tape Only." It was a shame that so many of the medical personnel couldn't read and continued to use the wrong tape, thought the Conselyeas.

Saturday, June 22
Day 41

Alysa very restless! H.R.=180's. Thrashing. 1:00 p.m. Given Morphine. 2:00 Dr. Otis began blood transfusion, 2 units. Temp normal. H. R.= 90's. Dave arrived at 5:00. Sylvia just left. Alysa resting peacefully since blood transfusion and Morphine.

Grandpa and Grandma Conselyea came to see her at 5:30.
B.P.=100/70. Still nice and calm. Given Versed because biting
tongue at 10:20. 11:45 Discontinuing Amphotericin. May be
causing rash. Given shot of Benadryl. 11:55 Temp=103. 1:15 a.m.
H.R.=107.

Linda walked into Alysa's room and discovered that she was having a blood transfusion. She nearly fainted!

"Please, tell me, what has happened? What is going on?" she demanded.

The nurse quickly explained. "Dr. Otis ordered a blood transfusion because your daughter's hemoglobin had dropped. Let's see...the chart says it's 6.7. Normal hemoglobin is 10."

"I don't understand. What causes hemoglobin to drop?"

"I'll let Dr. Otis explain that. I think he's still on the floor."

Linda paced the small quarters and fussed with the covers on Alysa's bed. Her agitation was noticeable to Dr. Otis as he came into the area.

"Mrs. Conselyea. You have a question?"

"Oh yes, Doctor. Thank you for coming so soon. Why does Alysa need a blood transfusion?"

"Her hemoglobin level is unusually low. It could mean that she has some internal bleeding, or it could be another reaction from the drugs. It seemed prudent in her vulnerable position to keep her blood level strong and healthy. She will receive two units; that's about a pint of blood. That should fix her up."

"I guess I overreacted. I was just shocked to see yet one more tube hooked up to Alysa. The poor thing," she said. "When she has a rash, she can't scratch it. She can't tell us how she feels. She can't cry tears. She can't make sounds. It seems so unfair," Linda finished, just shaking her head.

The doctor came over and put his arm around Linda. "We are going to find out what is wrong with her. In the meantime, we are going to keep her comfortable and strong. Don't you worry."

"Thank you, doctor. With all of you and with the great Physician, our Lord, she will get well. Sometimes I come unglued."

He flashed her a smile. "Well, I'll bring you some super glue, okay?"

Linda smiled back. "Okay. That would be nice."

"Hello, Mrs. Conselyea. We thought we'd come and see how Alysa was doing," Heidi Graunstadt said, as she and her husband Darren approached Alysa's bed. They were the owners of the L.A. Café in Waterford.

"Well, hello. It is so nice of you to come," Linda replied.

"How *is* she doing?"

"Not very well. The doctors are still not sure what's causing the seizures. Plus she has had additional infections and severe allergic reactions to the drugs. They are trying to treat her symptoms."

"Will she know it if I talk to her?" Darren asked.

"We don't know for sure, but please do say something. We talk to her all the time. It seems to comfort her and it makes us feel better."

He walked over to his former employee and tried not to look at the apparatus attached to Alysa. "Hey—Big Al. We sure could use you back at the coffee bar. No one has even come close to your expertise with mixing and blending the special coffees. Why don't you get well and we'll hire you back?"

The Graunstadts had taken Alysa under their wing when they first opened the restaurant. Alysa had served the gourmet coffees at her mom's candy shop, so she was experienced with the machines when she came to work for them.

"It's so hard to see her this way," Heidi said. "She was so full of energy and was always laughing. The regulars loved her. And she enjoyed joking and teasing them, too. Dougie, a guy who came in every day, still asks about her."

"I'm curious," Linda remarked. "How did she get the nickname Big Al?"

"Oh that," Darren said. "Big Al managed the coffee bar with an iron hand. She kept everyone, employee and customer alike, in line. No one wanted to mess with her. Actually, she was very polite and courteous with a little perverse humor thrown in. She made everything fun."

"I know that she really liked working there," Linda said.

Heidi agreed. "She met some friends who hung out there and would go out with them after work. Alysa attracted business."

They exchanged small talk with Linda, and then the pair left giving Alysa an awkward farewell.

Another MRI was scheduled on the 24th. Again, Alysa was given drugs to calm her movements. Going for the MRI was not an easy feat. She was wheeled down the hallway with a respiratory therapist hand "bagging" her the entire trip, with a back-up machine trailing along. The squeezing of the football-looking bulb was like a wooshing drumbeat.

The therapist kept the beat down the hall, into the elevator and into the MRI center in the annex. A special tubing reached into the MRI machine so that the bagging was uninterrupted. An MRI could last an hour or longer. A tag team of therapists kept the bag squeezing throughout the test.

Dave: "I am amazed at the medical knowledge we absorbed throughout Alysa's illness. I was fascinated by the special scan she had on June 25. First, blood was drawn and taken to a nuclear medicine facility off the hospital grounds. There they spun out her white blood cells and added a nuclear medicine, isotopes. The radioactive isotopes were mixed with her blood and re-injected into her body. The isotopes cling to the white cells that, as fighters of infection, go to any source of infection in the body from brain to toes.

"Alysa was then taken to the nuclear lab in the hospital for a scan of her entire body. The isotopes would clearly indicate any areas of infection that had been missed before. In her case, the scan showed no infection. The technicians waited four more hours and took her for a second scan. Still no infection. I later learned and was surprised that most of the medical staff had not known about this particular procedure. Again, it was a mixed blessing. We were pleased that there was no infection. The question remained: why was Alysa so sick?"

*   *   *   *   *

"I'm here to talk to you about a possible brain biopsy," Dr. Bubala announced to Linda with a purposeful and confident air. The tall, lean Austrian-born specialist acknowledged himself as an expert in the field of neurosurgery.

"Your daughter's most recent MRI shows three brain lesions: one on either side of the outer cortex and one on the left side, deep, in the basal ganglia area. This last area could be the culprit

61

causing the seizures."

"Doctor, we were told before that a biopsy would not provide enough yield for any determination," Linda said. "What has changed?"

Not fond of being challenged, the doctor became rude and offensive. "Look, I was called in merely to consult on the MRI's and to give my opinion for a possible biopsy. I'm not saying that I want to do it. In fact, from observing your daughter, I'm guessing she has mad cow's disease or equine disease. To perform surgery on her would put me in grave danger. An operating room would have to be shut down for minute re-sterilization. My staff could die. I might die. This disease is so fatal that everyone would be at risk. I have no desire to get a biopsy." He concluded huffily, "If, somehow, your daughter survives, she'll be a vegetable the rest of her life!"

Stunned. Dumbfounded. Incredulity seeped into every fiber of Linda's soul. How could he take away Alysa's entire life based on a 10-minute observation? He had not looked at her files or her records or even discussed the case with the other doctors.

Linda: "I chose not to write his diagnosis in the journal. His words were so negative, so degrading and so devastating that I didn't even relate the conversation to Dave. I didn't want to upset everyone who was currently caring for Alysa. Besides, I did not believe it. I took it to the Lord in prayer."

Alysa underwent another MRI. Later, Dr. Bubala strode in as if he had not exploded in a previous outburst and said, "Well, this is pretty amazing. All three of the lesions have shrunk. Lesions don't shrink. She must not have mad cow's disease. I could be convinced to do the biopsy without exposing myself or my staff to imminent danger."

"Doctor, I'm not going to be the one to convince you," Linda responded and turned away from him to continue brushing Alysa's hair.

*   *   *   *   *

The culminating events in Alysa's illness created a major turning point in Linda's life. Alysa had a very bad night. Her heart was racing between 155 to 180 beats a minute. Exhausted and spent, Linda had been trying to leave since 11:00 p.m.

"Honey, why don't you go on home to your mom's," Dave suggested. "I'll stay here and if there is any problem or complication, I'll call you immediately. Okay?"

"I just can't leave until her heartbeat is down to at least 130."

"Come here, let's pray."

They held hands and audibly prayed for Alysa's heartbeat to decrease. Linda cried, and prayed, and cried, and prayed. They didn't know why the Lord wasn't answering this particular prayer. Finally, at 1:00 a.m. she dragged herself to the parking lot to leave.

Linda: "That was the first time that I lost complete control. I wept and wept for what seemed like forever. The entire car shook with my sobbing. From the pain I had later, I think I bruised my sternum. Moms are supposed to be able to fix anything. I couldn't fix it. I couldn't help her. I loved her so much and I was powerless. I begged and pleaded with God to fix her for me. Then I realized that I hadn't fully given Alysa to him. I had to place her 100% into God's hands. I spent the next 35 minutes talking to God and I relinquished everything to him. Whatever he chose to do with our precious lamb was his will, not mine. I felt a great release. The burden had been lifted. I turned the ignition and made the five-minute drive to mom's and sleep."

The next evening Ken, Dave and Linda went to Sylvia's for dinner as they had done so many times. They were always booted out of ICU around dinnertime as the nurses wanted to tend to Alysa without diversion. Normally, all three would return for the evening. This time Linda decided to let Dave and Ken return without her.

Linda: "Mom was downstairs and I could hear the Bill Gaither gospel music from my Dad's video in the next room. I was in the bedroom where Dave and I were sleeping, Alysa's former bedroom. I closed the door and got on my knees to pray. No words came. I had forgotten how to pray. I couldn't think of anything to say. So, I tried just talking to God. Again, nothing. I started to sing children's Sunday school songs. I didn't know what else to do. Then I sang 'Beautiful Savior.' The words to 'Holy, Holy, Holy' softly started to pour from my mouth. I couldn't quit singing it. I heard a quiet voice say, 'You have to trust me.' Lord! I do trust you! Then the voice clearly said 'Alysa has to trust me, too.' Oh,

Lord, I know she trusts you.

"It was impossible to stop singing 'Holy, Holy, Holy.' My hands were tightly fastened on the sides of my head. I couldn't pull them away. I remained like that for 27 minutes; I knew precisely, because I had looked at the digital clock. I knew there was a presence in the room. In that time, God told me that Alysa would be okay if I trusted him and if she trusted him. Simultaneously my singing stopped and my hands were shaken loose from my head. I gently fell back on the floor. I smiled as my face searched for the presence in the room. I felt it. I sensed it. It was the most awesome experience of my life. I don't expect to ever encounter anything like that again."

Dave came home at midnight and Linda asked him to go for a walk. They quietly closed the door behind them and Dave asked, "What's up?"

"Dave, I'm going to tell you something that happened to me tonight. It is so unbelievable…and exciting," she said with a slight tremor in her voice. She proceeded to recount her experience with the living God.

"Do you believe me?" she asked her husband.

Wrapping his arms around her and holding her closely, he spoke earnestly into her ear.

"Of course I believe you. I am so thrilled for you and I am so humbled that God chose to give you peace. 'He who belongs to God hears what God says.' (John 8:47) 'My peace I give you,'" (John 14:27) Dave quoted.

They walked along the deserted neighborhood, hand in hand, back to the little house that the Lord had visited.

The next day, Linda awoke with conviction. She dressed with confidence and felt joyous. She had a mission. She knew in her heart that Alysa trusted the Lord, but she felt the urgency of confirming Alysa's belief. She approached Alysa, who seemed restless. Alysa's hands were normally in a clenched position. The nurses would put washcloths in her hands to protect them and prevent atrophy. Today, Alysa's left hand was clenching, but her right hand was open, flat.

Linda grasped that open hand and leaned over nearer to Alysa. "Sweetheart, I have to tell you what happened to me last night." She explained in detail her phenomenal experience. "Alysa, I must know and God must know if you trust him completely. If you trust the Lord, please squeeze my hand."

And she did.

"Oh, Alysa," Linda said as her eyes brimmed with tears. "The beginning of your healing has begun. Praise God in all his glory!"

That afternoon provided evidence of improvement. The result of a lumbar puncture was encouraging. There was only one white cell in the spinal fluid—the same analysis as a healthy person's.

Linda: "I could have done cartwheels down the hallway! I was just so excited. I knew that we had a long journey ahead, but I had the unwavering hope to keep me going. God had a mighty work to do and we were going to be his instruments. We might not always understand, but God's plan is perfect. His purpose is eternal. We have an awesome God."

CHAPTER SEVEN

Summers on Dixie Lake provided glimpses into heavenly realms. Peace, tranquility, shimmery cool water and palate-streaked sunsets reigned supreme. But the Conselyeas would not enjoy one sunset or even dangle a bare foot off the dock into the water. The summer of 1996 would be spent at Alysa's side.

Alysa celebrated Independence Day from the confines of her bed. Linda had moved the bed over to the window, hoping Alysa could see the fireworks displayed from a nearby park. Ken had gone up to northern Michigan where half the Detroit populace goes for the holiday; Linda and Alysa were all alone.

"Lysa, Honey," Linda said as she lay down on the bed next to Alysa. "Look out the window. Can you see the beautiful fireworks? Oh, look, there's a shower burst of red and green. And, ohhhh, there's a blue one that burst into little white flickering lights. And hear the bangs of the explosions? It's the Fourth of July, Lysa. You have always loved fireworks."

But the fireworks that year elicited no response from Alysa.

Tuesday, July 9
Day 58

12:20 p.m. Ken here. Alysa sleeping. H.R.=101. Looks hot (red face and arms). Nurse says she has been quiet all day. Started on new medication. Will move to room 416 within the hour. Will

66

have second liver and pelvis scan this afternoon: maybe discover pain source. 2:00 All set up in new room. Normal temp, BP=110/60. 4:00 Temp=99.7. 7:00 Alysa back in room after scan down in radiology. Results tomorrow. Ken and Dave moved out of room. Doctor in to talk about Phenobarb and Klonipin. Alysa very sedated, therefore, very still. Breathing therapist in at 7:40. 8:00 Benadryl. 8:45 Respiratory therapist did breathing treatment. Breaths per minute, 19. 9:30 Turned her. Given 10:00 meds. Alysa given 5 mg Morphine because she was a little restless. Can't have Versed, Ativan or Valium. Nurse Suzi here. Going to turn her. Moving legs, sticking out tongue. H.R.=130 at 11:20 p.m. Ken still here. Biting tongue ever since Morphine. 11:50 Doing better. H.R.=120. Stopped biting tongue. Coughing spell at 1:00 a.m. Suction lungs and mouth by therapist.

Alysa had graduated to a step-down unit on July 9. She was out of the ICU because she no longer needed the constant care and monitoring. Of course, a new location meant new nurses and aides who weren't familiar with the case. The burden of explanation fell to the family members. They were always present, always familiar with Alysa's progress—or lack of it—as detailed in the journal entries that kept them busy doing SOMETHING!

"Your daughter must be having a seizure," one nurse said with alarm.

"No, those movements are continual. She is not seizing," Linda explained.

"Sticking her tongue out like that is normal?"

"Yes, but when she bites it like she is starting to do, we need to protect her tongue. It's turning blue," Linda pointed out, searching for the bite block. Finding one with the personal items that had traveled down the hall from ICU, she inserted it into Alysa's mouth, not without difficulty.

Being in a regular hospital room brought certain merits. There was a telephone. Now Alysa and her caregivers were connected with the outside world. The phone rang—Uncle Marc from California. Linda put the receiver next to Alysa's ear.

"Hi, Alysa! How are you doing? I hear you're in a new room. We're all fine here. It's another beautiful, boring day in California. Diane and the boys send their love. You get well!"

Expecting no response, Linda grinned gratefully when Alysa lifted her arms up as if she wanted a hug from her Uncle Marc. Alysa was on the respirator when Marc called, but she was getting CPAP trials—times when her breathing would be assisted by a computerized machine. The head respiratory therapist, John, explained to Dave how it worked.

"Alysa has been relying on the ventilator to do her breathing. Actually, she has forgotten how to breathe by herself. We want her to relearn how to breathe. We connect this computerized monitor to her respirator and set how many times we want her to breathe per minute. If she initiates a breath, that's one less breath that the machine takes for her. If she fails to initiate the breath, then the machine breathes for her. This takes a lot of physical effort on her part. Her lungs can get exhausted because she hasn't exerted any effort. We will come in several times a day and hook her up to see how many breaths she can do on her own," he concluded.

"Is there any way to judge when she will be off the breathing equipment entirely?" Dave asked.

"I'm afraid not. In her case, if she is extremely restless or is running a fever, then we don't like to do the trials. We want her to be relaxed and quiet when we have breathing treatments. My staff is great. I think Al here will do just fine," he said, giving Alysa a nickname that all the therapists found endearing.

Linda: "We really liked John. He seemed to have a special affinity for Alysa. His son developed seizures at the age of 14, so he knew what it was like. He would hold her hand and encourage her breathing. 'Come on Al, you can do it. One more breath—just for me. That's my girl,' he would say."

At first, Alysa would breathe on her own for only two or three minutes, but as the trials continued, her breathing accelerated. She stayed connected to the machine and initiated breaths for up to two hours. When she had a six-hour CPAP trial, Dave thought they should celebrate. He smuggled in a Popsicle for Alysa as a reward.

"Here, Sweetie Pie, take a lick. Just don't tell the speech therapist. It's our little secret," he said affectionately.

Linda kept her friends and prayer partners up to date on Alysa's condition. After preliminary pleasantries and always asking for their own prayer concerns, Linda launched into her report.

"Oh, there are so many reasons to praise the Lord! Alysa is bathed and dressed every day and sits up in a chair. They've removed the heart monitor, and she is learning how to breathe on her own. But, she is getting Morphine for pain and for her restlessness, and Klonipin for seizures, Vancomycin for a blood bacterial infection and so many other medications, that she has developed a serious rash. She is bright red from head to toe. It looks like she has a severe sunburn. The heat just radiates from her body. She must be so uncomfortable. Please pray for the rash to subside, the infection to be cured and for Alysa to be comfortable. Thanks."

Those prayers were slowly answered. Ice packs and a cooling blanket were placed on Alysa to reduce the heat. The doctors didn't like to use the cooling blanket for very long periods of time because it could lower the body temperature too far. It could cause ice burns on the flesh and it masked the reason for the fever. So Grandma Rivers and Linda would keep applying cold, wet washcloths on Alysa's neck, under her arms and in her groin area. It was determined that the Vancomycin was the cause of the rash, but it was the only drug that could fight the blood infection. Administering steroids helped to curtail the effect of the rash. The infection finally cleared so that Alysa could enjoy short periods of comfort.

Dave: "Our shift routine was pretty set. Linda and sometimes her mom would come around 10:30 in the mornings. They would stay most of the day. I'd come in the early evening and generally stay the night. Ken came on his lunch hour and back again after work. He usually spent the night. Linda Two filled in. Often she took night duty, in the room with Alysa, so I could get some rest. We would update each person as our shift ended."

On the morning of July 11, Dave relieved an exhausted Linda Two. She recounted the night to Dave after his innocent, "How'd it go last night?"

"Don't ask! Alysa had a bad night. After her breathing treatment at 11:30, she coughed a lot. She was given Phenobarb at 3:15 a.m. and by 3:30 she was totally wild. She fought me, the nurses, and her tubes and wires—and she tried to get up. She got Valium at 5:30, but still had hard right-arm movement. She was sweating like crazy and was beet red with what looked like a heat rash. By 7:00 this morning, her eyes were closed, but she still had a lot of involuntary movement."

"Was she sticking her tongue in and out?" Dave asked. For some reason, this particular affliction bothered him tremendously.

"Yes, she was very active until 9:00. Then more Valium calmed her down."

Alysa had absolutely no control over her actions. They were a result of her illness and her medications. To see her physically flailing her limbs with eyes wide open disconcerted her family and friends. With that much movement it was difficult to comprehend that she had no mental acuity. She continued to be out of touch with reality.

Dave nodded toward his daughter. "How long has she been sitting in the chair?"

"Since 9:35. Well, I'm beat. I'm heading out of here."

Dave put an arm around Linda Two. "There's no way I can thank you enough for your sacrifice to help us. You are one terrific lady, Linda."

"Yeah. You probably say that to all the girls who spend the night wrestling with Alysa."

"I wish," Dave said. "Take care."

When his wife arrived that morning, Dave related Alysa's night to her, adding, "Alysa is restless now. Her temp is normal, for a change, and her heart rate is 130. The wound nurse was in to check on Alysa's foot sores. She's ordering Batravan."

"Is that a topical ointment or another stupid oral drug?"

"It's topical—I think. The Lord knows she doesn't need another drug. I'm planning to go to the office at noon. I've got some houses to show at 1:00."

"Fine. I'll hold down the fort. I hope your client makes up his mind soon."

"Yeah, me, too."

That night when Dave and Ken arrived, it was Linda's turn to give Alysa's report.

"Alysa had two CPAP's (computerized breathing) today: one from 1:00 to 2:00 and another from 4:15 to 4:45. Her temp was up to 101.6 but now it is 100.3. Dr. Abraham was in and talked about getting her off the respirator again."

"We've heard that before," Ken said. "I wish they'd just do it."

"I know. Maybe since she is finally making progress, this time it will work."

Thus, the cycle continued. All that changed, day to day, were the degrees of temperature, the heart rate, the number of breaths per minute and the list of medications given. Add the various doctors and nurses and the different tests ordered and Alysa's medical activities were enumerated.

Although the activities and reports were clinical, never for a moment did anyone forget that a human soul was at stake. Alysa's life and her dignity garnered the utmost attention.

*   *   *   *   *

Pastor Jim and his wife Carol came to visit Alysa and to pray for her. Dave had the TV tuned to the Atlanta Summer Olympics with the sound turned down. He switched it off when they entered. Jim convinced the parents to go to lunch with them.

"Alysa is pretty agitated today," Dave said. "I hate to do it, but I'll have to restrain her hands while we're gone. Otherwise, she'll pull out her tubes." He lashed his daughter's hands to the bed rails

"I'm sorry, Sweetie, but it's for your own good. We'll be back in a little while."

Turning to Jim and Carol, Linda said, "I want to tell the nurses that we're leaving. It'll take just a minute."

They drove to the Country Inn. The featured special was fish and skins—a variation on the fish and chips theme. During their lunch, Linda told her pastor about her experience of hearing a voice that told her that Alysa would be healed.

"In the Bible, God never spoke to people the same way twice. The presence you felt and the voice you heard were truly from the Lord," he said, validating her experience.

That night, while watching TV in the hospital, they learned of the bombing of Olympic Park in Atlanta. Before they left Alysa's room, along with their nightly prayer for her, they included in their prayers those in Atlanta who had need of solace.

Interview with Pastor Jim Combs

The braces on his teeth and the casual jeans he wears enhance Pastor Jim Combs' youthful looks. In five minutes of conversation, Jim's daily goal is revealed: to see God's hand moving in his life and in the lives of his church members. His shorthand for it is "seeing God."

Here's how he describes seeing God in Alysa's illness:

I've learned how incredible it is to see God. If I don't ever see God's hand again in my life, I've had my share through this experience with Alysa and her family. Very few people can relate to how she was in the beginning. Only a handful who saw her then can comprehend the scope of what happened to her. But first, I want to tell you about Linda and Dave Conselyea.

It is my opinion that the more you love your mate and your children, the closer you become to God. Dave and Linda possess a great passion for each other, one that isn't always evident in a marriage. Their love for each other vibrates, and they shower that love on their daughter. Dave has always been Alysa's "real" dad, and to Alysa, he's "Dad."

I have a Master's degree in psychology. Let me tell you, a stress trauma like the one the Conselyeas experienced either makes a relationship better...or worse. Usually, it's worse. Mates leave. Divorce is rampant. Linda and Dave leaned on each other; their relationship grew stronger. Both of the Conselyeas have servant hearts. Linda was always a strong prayer warrior, but now she has developed a prayer lifestyle. She has discovered how real prayer is and how powerful her God is. Dave has often blessed the congregation with his outstanding singing voice, but the amazing blessing is how they impacted every nurse and every doctor they met, and every hospital and nursing home they entered.

Their family was not the first I've known to face extreme pain, but it is the first time I saw a family react the way they did. Over a great period of time, they stood the test. They went through the Job thing, where others suggested they "curse God and die." Their faith never wavered. Their personal pain became overwhelming at times, but they were never hopeless.

At the beginning, Linda brought Alysa to the church for the elders to pray for her. Alysa had been feeling strange. We laid our hands on her and prayed for her victory in the spiritual battle. Afterwards, Greg Thomas, one of my staff, commented to Alysa, "God must be ready to so do something pretty incredible with you." What an understatement!

What Alysa endured at the beginning of her hospitalization

was the most unbelievable thing I've seen in my twenty years as a minister. The convulsions, the seizures, her eyes rolling back in her head, her jerking: all sickened me. As her physical and mental trauma increased and heightened throughout those months, the world's view labeled her useless: permanently prone, immobile and mute. Wrong. She was still God's child.

Another time in the hospital we again were praying for Alysa. I was holding her hand. While others prayed, I felt connected to Alysa. It was absolutely a spiritual reaction. I could feel the presence of the enemy. It was a full out attack on Alysa. The fury of Hell was lashed against her for some reason. The devil thought he had won that day, but the longer I prayed for Alysa, the tighter her hand squeezed. Satan tugged on her life, but with a mom and dad who wanted to see God, he didn't have a chance.

When the doctors came to a dead end and said they knew nothing more to do, and they knew no one else in the country with the answers, that was a good starting place for God.

I'm not surprised by the grace of God. There were hundreds and hundreds of people praying for Alysa every day. My three-year-old son, Luke, kept Alysa's picture on the refrigerator and prayed for her "to get well." The picture showed Lysa with the trache tube in her throat. He didn't understand the machine, but he learned what God is all about. We have an incredible Savior, Jesus, through whom we pray.

One of the saddest things the unbeliever misses out on is the power of prayer. Having a positive attitude does help the psyche, but setting our mind on the knowledge that God works in our lives is life changing. Only a fraction of believers have the tiniest concept of prayer. Prayer is the most needed aspect of the believer's life and the most neglected. We have yet to tap this transforming tool that God has given us.

Alysa's story has touched every member of our congregation. They embrace God's faithfulness to his people through prayer. Dave and Linda taught me about faith.

Interview with Sylvia Rivers

A little, gray, barking schnauzer greets everyone at the door of the Rivers' house. Heidi eagerly sniffs each newcomer only to be disappointed if it isn't Alysa. With the constant traffic of family and friends, that's a lot of sniffing. The Rivers have stretched their open-door policy to that of a revolving door.

As Sylvia tells it:

I came from a very loving Christian family of twelve children. We were extremely close and we knew that we were loved. Family was the most important thing in our lives, and it still is to me. My family comes first, no matter what.

Andy and I have five children: Mike, Linda, Carol, Marc and Vicki. Both of the boys live in California so we don't get to see them very often. Marc and Diane have three adopted sons, now. Since I'm already caring for two of my grandchildren, plus Alysa when she was here, I've threatened to mail my California grandsons back if they show up in the mailbox one of these days. Vicki is divorced but has recently remarried and has two sons, Billy and Sean. She works in a doctor's office. Carol recently married Jim Klott and they live nearby. We have supported all of our children through the good times and the bad.

Our home was a haven for Linda more than once. She and her first husband lived here when she was first married. After Alysa was born, Linda returned to work and I took care of the baby. Linda's husband was lazy and had no real means of support. He was selfish and self-centered and thought we could provide whatever the baby needed.

Alysa was a bold child. At age four she would walk up to a total stranger who was smoking and say, "You're going to die." She loved watching the cheerleaders on television. She would constantly mimic them, doing her cheers all around the house.

When she moved here in 1995, to be close to school and work, it was really fun. She was so easy to talk to. She was so out-going and happy. She'd come home and tell me about her day. Sometimes she'd help cook dinner and often she would help the boys with their homework. Then she started feeling bad. Her behavior became so strange that I knew something was wrong. In retrospect, we should have taken her to a doctor, but nothing seemed to be of great significance at the time.

After my daughter Vicki's divorce a few years ago, I kept her two children for her after school and in the summers. I probably wouldn't choose to watch the children, but the circumstances are that I am needed. Besides, Billy and Sean are good boys.

When Alysa was hospitalized, it did not seem unusual to have Linda and Dave move in with us so they could be near the hospital. That's what families are for. After that first week, someone stayed with Alysa 24 hours a day. We read the Bible to her every day and none of us left the room without praying for her and telling her we loved her.

We learned what is important in life and what isn't. We also trusted in the Lord. God is who he says he is and he will do what he says. "Do not be afraid or discouraged...for the battle is not yours, but God's." I was never angry at God because I knew that God was taking care of her. As problems would arise in Alysa's care, we would ask Linda what, specifically, did she want us to pray about. Linda would tell us, "seizures, no pneumonia, comatose state, speech, breathing, eating," whatever was needed at the time. Our entire church was praying for her and many of us were fasting.

Andy and I prayed and fasted every Monday and Thursday and we have continued to do so. We won't eat from dinnertime on Sunday to dinnertime on Monday and again on Wednesday to Thursday. The entire experience has made us stronger. We are closer to each other and closer to the Lord. God always has a purpose and he allowed Alysa to become ill. It has been a blessing to a lot of people, probably more than we will ever know.

Interview with Andy Rivers
The tall, angular, Canadian-born Andrew Rivers is known as "Poophead" by his adoring granddaughter, Alysa. That was the worst thing she could ever think of to call him when, as a young adult in their home, she got mad at her grandfather for fussing at her to clean her room. He wears that and many other titles proudly: faithful husband, hard worker, strong father, loving grandfather, and faithful believer.

In Andy's words:
After my parents divorced when I was six-and-a-half, I was passed around to various aunts and uncles. My background was as unstable as Sylvia's was solid. Catholic boarding schools became my poor substitute for family. When I was only 17, I slipped over the border, changed my name from Lariviere to Rivers, lied about my age and joined the service.

Stationed in Japan for 39 months, I was a staff sergeant in the 35th Air Police. Right after I arrived, I got a "Dear John" letter from my girlfriend. Then I was called into the office and was chewed out by my commanding officer. He said I had four men in my squadron of eighteen men who were not writing letters home. I was to keep their passes until they wrote letters. One of those passes belonged to Sylvia's brother. Ken, a good friend of mine, found writing pure agony. He labored through four lines and then quit. I had some photos I'd taken of the two of us, so I asked if he'd mind if I jotted a few lines and threw in a picture or two. He was all for it! I got a letter in return from his sister. We wrote to each other for five months. Some of my letters were getting pretty mushy. She went to Cincinnati, met a sailor and got married on me. That's while my mushy letters were still in transit.

Next thing you know, I started getting letters from another of Ken's sisters, Sylvia. We wrote to each other for thirty-one months. I asked Ken if he thought Sylvia would accept a ring in the mail and then if we met and it didn't work out, we'd call it off. "What's to lose?" he said. So Sylvia and I became engaged sight unseen. Pretty romantic, huh?

I returned stateside on December 21, and on the 24th arrived in North Carolina where Sylvia's family lived. We got blood tests and were married at 12:15 on Christmas Day, 1951. It must have been right, because our 46th wedding anniversary is coming up.

We moved to Michigan, and I hired in at General Motors. I eventually became a molding engineer at the General Motors Tech Center, and I retired from that position on March 1, 1993. We've lived in this little house since 1985 and we've seen joys and heartaches. I had been shown Catholicism in my youth, but not until after I was married did I become saved and know Jesus Christ.

With my experience as a kid, I hated divorce, but I was relieved when Linda divorced her first husband. Alysa was God's blessing from that union.

Alysa was a determined little girl—took after her grandpa! When she was just a little tyke, about fourteen months old, she loved to go outside and smell the flowers and look at the tulips. If it was too hot for her, she just removed her clothing. She'd be naked as a jay bird, free as could be, admiring those flowers.

She liked helping her grandpa. We had a load of horse manure delivered for those same flower beds. I had to wheel it from the driveway to the gardens. She pitched in and helped. Was she ever a mess when we were finished.

When Sylvia was out, I'd get Alysa up on my lap and we'd read her favorite story books. We gave her her very own children's Bible. Sylvia made a lot of Alysa's clothes, especially for Sunday best. We'd take that little darling to church with us. She carried her little Bible and was so proud. I guess we more or less spoiled her.

When she got sick, I was devastated. I didn't understand why it couldn't have been me instead. The first several days were really hard for me. What helped me to overcome my grief and anger was to watch and listen to Bill Gaither videos. One was entitled "Sing Your Blues Away." The words from "Joy Comes In The Morning" brought me great comfort:

"To invest your seed of trust in God, in mountains you cannot move, you have risked your life on things you cannot prove, but to give up things you cannot keep, for what you cannot use. Now that's the way to find the joy God has for you.

"So, hold on my child, joy comes in the morning, weeping only lasts for the night. Hold on child, joy comes in the morning, the darkest hour means dawn is just in sight."

People are ministered to in different ways. With some, it's the scriptures. To someone else it might be a sermon or the encouraging words of a pastor. For me, listening to God's words and promises through those songs brought comfort.

Dave and I would go down in the family room, pop in the video and crank up the volume real loud. We were both touched by the lyrics and we shed a lot of tears. I kept retreating to those videos for solace. One day when I was home alone, I got mad and I had to let it out. I yelled, I mean really screamed, to God. What do you want me to do? You healed the blind. You took care of the woman who had been bleeding for 12 years. What are you going to do with Alysa?

Then I realized that I wasn't the one in control. Alysa was in his hands and he was going to take care of her in his own time. I learned how to wait. It was an enormous lesson for me. It was then that I attended a seminar with about 20 others from our church. "Fasting for Spiritual Breakthrough" was the topic, based on the book by Dr. Elmer Towns. In a nutshell, I learned to wait, fast, pray, accept what happens and rely on God. Not myself. It turned things around for me.

Sylvia and I adopted that attitude and discipline and we grew spiritually. It seemed like a blanket was being knit around us and we were all drawn in close. That got us through the rough times.

One time in particular was pretty bad for me. After Alysa got transferred to Oakhill Memorial, we went to see her. She didn't know us. She was on that ventilator machine and she was comatose but making those horrible jerking motions. We didn't yet know her diagnosis. The pain and the heartache of seeing her like that, my only granddaughter, is indescribable. I just stood there and cried. I had to go heavy on the videos after that visit. And I had to wait, and fast and pray.

CHAPTER EIGHT

A flicker of Alysa's independence glimmered the next day. She decided she preferred to lie sideways across the bed. Her position posed a predicament for the nurses. Nursing supervisors liked to see the patients neat and tidy with the sheet pulled up. A well-tucked patient meant a well-cared-for patient.

"Alicia's driving us crazy today," Nurse Sally said. "We keep re-positioning her, and she moves back like this," she gestured with disdain to Alysa, who had her legs hanging over the side of the bed.

"First of all, her name is pronounced Uh-lee-suh," Linda said.

"Alicia, Alysa, they sound the same to me."

"I can assure you they don't sound the same to her. She hates it when her name is mispronounced. One of her high school teachers never got it right. She kept correcting him and his response was 'Whatever.' She was furious."

"Okay, I got it. Uh-lee-suh."

"Good. Now, tell you what..." said Linda as she lowered the side rails on the bed, "Why don't we just humor her? I'm going to lie down beside her and read to her."

Sally glanced at the book and asked, "What are you reading to her?"

"Oh, it's one of Janette Oke's books: *Love's Abiding Joy*, about a family on a ranch in the Canadian plains whose lives are shattered by a tragic accident and...."

"Give me a love story with passion any old day. I don't want to read about tragedy. There's enough of that around here."

"That's true. But we can always learn about coping when we see how someone else does it—especially if that someone relies on the Lord."

The nurse made no further comment and left the room. In the hall she spoke to another nurse. "Her mom insists that I pronounce her daughter's name right. Big deal. She wouldn't know if I called her Anastasia."

Linda turned to Alysa, the "rebel." "Let's see where we left off yesterday. Here we are, page 202." With excitement in her voice, Linda began reading about the young man who placed his hope in his teacher instead of the Lord, and why following a man can only bring disappointment.

Alysa seemed content. The cadence of her mother's reading reassured her. She continued in her rebellious posture until she knew no one was going to move her. Linda chose this as a good time to deliver a pep talk.

"Alysa, you need to get off the respirator. Are you afraid to go off of it?"

Amazingly, Alysa nodded her head, "Yes."

Encouraged, Linda pursued her questioning, "Are you willing to trust God to help you? He'll help you if you are willing to try."

Tears of relief, frustration or perhaps fear fell from Alysa's dark eyelashes and onto her pillow. Obviously determined and comprehending, she disconnected the respirator herself. Linda had not expected immediate compliance and wasn't sure of the correct procedure, so at first, she reconnected the machine. Alysa unhooked it again. Linda connected it. It happened a third time. The phone rang.

"Oh, Dave. I'm glad it's you. Alysa is awake— praise God!— and I asked her if she wanted to get of the respirator and she keeps unhooking it. I told her that we wanted her to stop depending on it, and she just turned it off. She seems determined."

"Well, why don't you go for it? What's the worst thing that can happen? You can always connect her again. Maybe she's ready to make the step on her own."

"I just want her to be safe, but if she disconnects it one more time, I think we'll just leave it off. Pray for us!"

Linda closed the door. She felt as if she were doing something clandestine. "Dear Lord, let this be of your doing. Help Alysa to breathe on her own; give her this victory and let her know that you are her strength. Thank you Lord, for your love and your mercy. In Jesus' name, Amen."

Linda tensely watched her daughter breathe successfully. One long hour into her time off the respirator, Dave came in carrying a pizza.

"She's still off!" he exclaimed.

"Yes, it's been an hour now. She's doing it! God is so good."

Dave held the machine up to the trache hole in Alysa's neck and noted her oxygen level and her breaths per minute. "It looks great," he told Linda.

They celebrated with a hug and a kiss...and pepperoni pizza.

Joyce, one of the respirator therapists, made her normal rounds to check on Alysa. She was very surprised, but pleased, to find her patient unhooked. She checked the readings. "I hear nothing. I see nothing. I know nothing," she said as she backed out of the room. But then, she kept returning to check on and encourage Alysa.

Three hours later, Dave couldn't contain his excitement.

"This is just unbelievable. What an answer to prayer! Her heart rate is 93, her oxygen level is 96 and she is taking 17 breaths per minute. This is wonderful, just wonderful."

At 11:30 that night as often happened, Alysa got excited when Ken came into the room. It was necessary to put her back on the ventilator to calm her down.

Her trial and her trust did not go in vain. On Sunday as Linda parked her car in the hospital parking lot, one of the employees saw her and greeted her enthusiastically.

"Hey, Mrs. Conselyea! Have you heard the good news? Alysa is going to get off the respirator tomorrow! Dr. Burke wrote the order. Isn't that great?"

A knowing smile spread on Linda's face. "It most certainly is. It's wonderful news."

And that's what happened.

On day number 78 of Alysa's hospital stay, the respiratory therapist, John, came into Alysa's room. Alysa had been on the respirator for 60 days.

He went to her bedside and sat down beside her. "Hi, Al. This is your big day. You've graduated. We're going to take the ventilator away. You're improving so much, next thing you know, you'll be eating steak and lobster. Let's just hope the cafeteria doesn't fix it, right?" he said jokingly, patting her on the shoulder. As he wheeled the machine out the door, he reassured her, "I'm still going to come in every day and check on my girl, okay?"

"Alysa, I'm so happy. Let's call your grandma and tell her the good news, want to?" Linda dialed the number. "Mom, it's Linda. Lysa is off the vent. It's been taken out of the room. Why don't you come up and see for yourself? Okay, see you in a little while."

Sylvia arrived shortly, Sean with her. "Hi, Lys," Sean greeted his cousin. "How ya' doin'?"

Alysa seemed to direct her attention to her cousin. Not always cognizant of those around her, her awareness seemed heightened. Recognition registered in slow motion.

She smiled at her grandmother and her cousin.

"Hi, Sweetheart," Sylvia said as she smoothed Alysa's hair around her thinning, pale face. "I'm so thrilled you're off the respirator. You're getting better. Thank the Lord!"

That night Alysa slept through the entire night for the first time since her illness began.

As with most mountaintop highs, a valley low often follows. Bacteria again attacked Alysa's blood. That meant the dreaded Vancomycin with its accompanying rashes and extreme distress. This time, perhaps a steroid would lessen the drug's effect.

Many strides were made the next day. The occupational therapist elicited a full range of motion on Alysa's arms, albeit in slow motion. The speech therapist offered Alysa baby food peaches from a sponge. She gave Linda instructions.

"If you want to try to give her some applesauce tonight, you may. And if you think she is trying to say something, let me show you what to do. Just take your fingers and close off the hole in her trache. That should help you to distinguish sounds and speech."

The Phenobarbital hindered Alysa's mental and physical reactions. She would try to do what the therapists asked, but responded in delayed, deadened movements. Dr. Abraham, Alysa's favorite physician, and the head nurse were consulting in Alysa's room when she desperately wanted to show Dr. Abraham what she had learned in O.T. Foggily, she painstakingly raised her arms, repeating her therapy exercises. Frustrated with her own inability to perform for him, tears welled and spilled down her cheeks. Realizing that his patient was working hard just to please him, Dr. Abraham, caught off guard, began to cry and had to excuse himself from the room.

*   *   *   *   *

Monday, August 5
Day 85

Dave writing entry. Linda gave Alysa bath and shaved legs and armpits. She stood on her own two legs when nurse went to put her in chair at 10:45. Pat, Becky, and Christy Toth and Pat Thomas came to visit. Went down to lunch at 12:45. Dr. Owens came in—Alysa performed with concentration. Very pleased! Dr. Abraham in. Alysa closed her eyes until he left. Dr. Baker in, says 3-4 days on Vancomycin. Back in bed at 4:30. Very comfortable. Grandma Rivers here 5:30. Noticed after Klonopin, head stiff and eye movement. Lasted about 15 minutes. Linda C. left at 6:00. Temp= 98. Dave came in at 10:00. Grandma Rivers and Ken here. G'ma R left at 10:15. Alysa's feeding tube came out. Kelly, nurse, and Linda Two who came in at 10:30 changed bed. Alysa pulled out Foley catheter again (twice today). Otherwise, she's doing well. Linda Two spending night tonight. Linda Two writing. 12:30 Breathing treatment and night meds. 1:00 a.m. to 1:30 a.m. Sat up in bed. Very active. Settled down with both legs over rail and crossed, sideways in bed. Went to sleep till 2:00 a.m. Active. Trying to cough. Phenobarb at 3:00 a.m. 4:00 a.m. Advil and breathing treatment. 4:30 Very active. 5:30 Temp=101. 6:45 a.m. Meds. Calmed down. Dr. Abraham at 7:15.

Mastering her arm movements, Alysa performed for Dr. Owens, one of her neurologists, when he came in to see her.

"This is just fantastic! Alysa, you are doing so well." Turning to Linda, he said, "This definitely is a good sign. I think we're on the right road. Dr. Sandy Silverton is the director of the area's rehabilitation centers. I'm going to give her a call and have her evaluate Alysa. That may be our next step."

Pat Toth and her daughters and Pat Thomas visited just before lunch. They all greeted Alysa and as women will, starting chattering. The tape "Standing Together" by Homeward Bound competed to be heard from the windowsill tape player. It lost.

A few days later, Dr. Silverton conducted her evaluation. She was a kind, gentle woman who was extremely patient with Alysa. She noted that Alysa could make some movements on command, that she could sit in the chair and that she was capable of eye contact and comprehension.

On August 12, Alysa laughed and smiled with Dr. Abraham!

The scripture that Dave read to Alysa that night was Jeremiah 17:14. "Heal me. O Lord, and I will be healed; save me and I will be saved, for you are the one I praise."

Alysa shook her head up and down. She was in total agreement.

Pointing to his own blonde locks, Dave teased his daughter.

"Look at what you've done to me. I'm beginning to look like a Hippie. You have to hurry up now and get well so you can give me a haircut. Dad is starting to complain. I refuse to get it cut until you can do it, you hear? I'll wait for you."

Good events snowballed. Alysa was trying to talk. A "talking trache" was fitted so sounds could be amplified. Alysa was making appropriate facial expressions. Her chest X-ray was clear—no pneumonia. She spoke! Her words were "no," "no," "no, don't," "don't." The source of her frustration was unknown, but they were recognizable words!

Code Blue! It happened in a second. Alysa was getting prepped for a CAT scan. The nurse, Diane, glanced at Alysa and saw that she was not breathing. "Blue" was called to the House Officer and respiratory ward. Every nurse and doctor on the floor came running into the room. A crash cart was rushed in. Alysa coughed. She coughed again. A mucous plug appeared. The emergency was over. Alysa regained her color, but she remained wide-eyed.

"Alysa, were you frightened?" Diane asked.

"Yes." A new word.

"Well, it's over now. You were able to cough that up and get it out. That's my girl. Just relax. You're going to be okay now," she continued, soothingly. Everyone else filed out of the room, with relief etched on their faces.

84

Linda approached Alysa with her arms outstretched. Alysa lifted her arms to her mother.

"Here I am, Lys. Let me hold you, Honey," she said as she gathered her to her chest.

Alysa returned the hug. The CAT scan was postponed. With the uttering of motherly comfort and calming, the two fell asleep entwined.

*　　*　　*　　*　　*

"Head hurts," Alysa said clearly to Elaine, startling the nurse who was changing her bedding.

"What? Did you say something, Alysa?"

"Head hurts."

"Well, let's take care of that." She prepared an ice pack for the back of Alysa's neck.

"Now, I'm going to have the doctor order some Toridol for you right away. That will take care of your headache."

Elaine collided with Linda in the doorway. "Alysa told me her head hurts. She talked! I'm on my way down to the pharmacy myself to get her some Toridol."

Linda rushed into the room. She had been gone for only fifteen minutes, but that was long enough to miss her daughter's first coherent comment in 11 weeks.

Linda had been visiting with Alysa's Great Grandmother Bisson, Andy's mother, who had been admitted to Room 606 on the oncology floor the day before, her bladder cancer in advanced stages.

"So, Sweetie, you have a bad headache?" she asked while stroking her daughter's cheek.

"Yes."

"Elaine has gone to get you something. I'm so glad that you can tell us where you hurt, Alysa. It is wonderful to know exactly what's the matter so we can help you to feel better."

Linda talked to her daughter just as she had before but now, she knew, Alysa could hear and respond. "Great Grandma Bisson is upstairs. She asked about you and said for you to get well. Grandma and Grandpa Rivers are with her. They'll be down in a little while."

A good day was followed by a bad night.

Monday, August 19
Day 99

Dad here. Hasn't stayed still for more than five minutes. Gets the sweats. Jenny sponging her off. From 12:30 to 2:30 a.m. all over the bed. Dave held her legs from jerking for approximately five minutes. She hasn't moved them in over 20-30 minutes. Jenny went to get Toridol per my request. Given at 2:45. Drug had no effect. Alysa going through what appears to be epileptic motions. It goes from severe to mild to severe again. Total lack of muscle control. She has been going through HELL tonight. I only wish I could help her.

Because of Linda Two's own tenuous health, and her Lupus diagnosis, her physician had ordered her off night duty for the Conselyeas. Dave now took the full responsibility to be with Alysa during the dark hours of the night.

Dave: "If someone weren't with Alysa all the time, she would be tied up in restraints. We hated that. For some reason, her condition seemed to worsen at night and in the early hours of the morning. I remember one such night in mid-August. It was horrible to watch. Alysa twisted her body as if she were a professional contortionist. With closed eyes she stretched her neck and tried to rotate her head. The top half of her body lunged in one direction, and the bottom half turned the opposite way. Her arms bent at awkward angles in back of her. I couldn't bear her apparent agony. After an hour or two of watching her gyrate, I had to intervene—both verbally and physically.

"I took her arms and legs and forced them down on the bed. That night I even lay down on top of her, trying not to put all of my weight on her thinning body. She was so strong! She aggressively fought my attempts to quiet her. I just wanted her to be still—for her to have a moment's peace and rest. It was not to be.

"Discouraged, depressed and frustrated I prayed for the demons inside this girl to leave her alone. I didn't know if those demons were the virus, the drugs or the seizures, but something sinister was affecting her system. I felt so helpless. I didn't know what to do anymore. We had prayed for instantaneous healing. The answer was no. We can't make someone else be still. The Holy Spirit prepares our hearts. 'Be still and know that I am God.'

I could not still Alysa. But I knew God could and would."

*   *   *   *   *

After that horrendous night with Alysa, Dave decided not to cancel his long-planned golf outing coming up in early September. Time away would be restoration to his soul. Besides, golf was his avocation.

Alysa had several agitated, restless days in a row. Ken had arrived at 5:30 after work to find Alysa emerging from a brief sleep. Dave and Linda were having a rare dinner out with her sister Carol and Jim Klott at the Outback Steakhouse. After her medications and breathing treatment, Alysa returned to a peaceful sleep. Carrie, Ken's sister, brought him fried rice for his dinner, which he thoroughly enjoyed. He wrote in the journal, "Alysa still sleeping. (PTL). I'm sounding like Dave!" Nurse Toni bustled in.

"Alysa hasn't really slept for three days. Please don't disturb her right now, okay?"

Ken thought she was going to check the Foley catheter when she raised the sheet, but instead she changed Alysa's sleeping position and moved her legs onto the bed.

"What are you doing?" Ken asked, contemplating strangling the nurse.

Startled, she left the room in a huff. Alysa stirred a little, but appeared to go back to sleep. Peaceful body status was so rare, that no one wanted Alysa disrupted when it occurred. When the nurse returned at 9:30 to take vitals, Ken asked, politely, if she could wait until Alysa were awake.

"Fine. Let me know when she's awake."

Alysa awoke at 9:50. She moved her arms and made gurgling sounds. She scrunched up her face but didn't seem to be having seizures. Next, she touched her face with her fingertips, as if it were an object of delicate but unfamiliar origin.

Alysa had her trache capped. With the opening closed, speech was greatly facilitated. One day, she said tentatively, "Ly-sa. Ly-sa. Ly-sa." Joy was abundant in room 416 that day!

On August 29th, the day before Alysa's birthday, the trache apparatus was completely removed from Alysa's throat. Alysa's reaction was to cry. And Dave and Linda joined in. Her oxygen level remained at 95. Perfect. What a nice birthday present.

Hospital rooms rank low on the list of popular venues for celebrating birthdays, but the Conselyeas were not deterred. August 30, 1996, Alysa Conselyea turned 22, and nearly everyone in the hospital knew it.

Showing up early in the day were Pat, Christy, and Becky Toth along with Carolyn Mack. They brought cards, and Christy presented Alysa with a back massager from Body Works. Carrie and Matt, Ken's sister and brother, popped in with an entire bag full of clothes from all the Komisarz. Nikki had added waffle weave boxers and a matching top. There were fashionable pants and shirts for the stylish hospital patient.

Aunt Carol arrived at lunchtime with a card and best wishes. Linda Two called to give her regards to the birthday girl and so did Leslie from Social Services. The Physical Therapy and Occupational Therapy departments gave Alysa a big, brown, cushy stuffed bear.

Sylvia had done the culinary honors and brought for the occasion a dark chocolate torte plus a banana cake with white chocolate shavings. After the presentation of the cake and the singing of "Happy Birthday," Linda and Dave mounted the cakes on a hospital cart and wheeled it around to all of their favorite nurses and doctors on the fourth and fifth floors.

Their popularity with the staff grew proportionately to the pieces of cake distributed. They took some to Grandma Bisson on six and then to Grandpa Rivers on the third floor. He had been admitted the day before for prostate surgery. Aunt Karen, Dave's sister, rounded out the guest list that afternoon. The birthday girl heard the birthday refrain whenever someone came into her room. She probably thought it was a broken record. With friends and family all around, it wasn't such a terrible birthday after all.

Alysa was kidnapped the next day. Kelly, Ken's sister, came to visit. Alysa was sitting in a reclining chair that Linda had been pushing through the hallways to give Alysa different scenery and to reintroduce her to lights, sounds and people. They met Kelly at the end of the hallway.

"Hi, Alysa. You going for a ride?" she asked her brother's girlfriend.

Lysa's eyes were open, but she didn't respond to the question. Linda answered, "That room gets stale and boring. I thought it would do Alysa some good to get out of there and look around."

"It's a gorgeous day. Why don't we take her outside?" Kelly suggested.

"That's an intriguing idea." Linda glanced around at the personnel in the hall on the fourth floor. Most seemed preoccupied and were not paying attention to the trio. Linda started inching toward the elevator with her co-conspirator by her side. She pushed the down button and the elevator doors jumped open. They made their escape, carefully loading the chair onto the elevator. The doors closed. So far, so good.

They exited on ground level and acted very purposeful and official. They pushed their captive out the door and into the sunshine. Freedom! No people milled around or looked at them suspiciously. The heat of the day shocked their air-conditioned skin. The pungent aroma of hot asphalt mixed with freshly cut grass filled their nostrils.

Linda: "It was exhilarating. It felt good to be alive. But we had to soothe Alysa because she was frightened and unsure about her surroundings. I took off her booties and placed her bare feet on a small patch of grass. The unusual sensation brought some glimmer of recognition to her face."

"I think she likes it," Kelly said.

"Well, I sure do. She hasn't been outdoors for over three and a half months."

"The sun feels pretty good, too, don't you think, Lys?"

Lys said nothing to her friend.

"How could you do that to me?" Dr. Raines said the next day when Linda confessed to the previous day's outing. "I was working in the emergency center yesterday. I wasn't even available!"

"I knew where you were and how to get there if there were problems," she reassured him. "Besides, the risk was worth it to get fresh air, hear the birds, feel the grass and see the sun. We survived," she reminded him.

*   *   *   *   *

Linda, on the other hand, needed more than a change of scenery. With three members of her family in the hospital all at the same time, she felt stretched beyond her capabilities.

Linda: "It was not a fun time. I was on the verge of losing it.

And to top it all off, Judy Slone, Traumatic Brain Injury System Co-ordinator, from the Detroit Medical Center Rehabilitation Institute of Michigan came to assess Alysa for her admittance to a rehabilitation facility. A patient is graded on a scale from zero to eight. A score of three is needed to enter rehab. Alysa barely passed receiving a four. We then had to wait for approval.

"We were turned down. We weren't told why, but we think it was because of insurance. In a disappointed and despondent mood, I improved after getting phone calls from friends and family. God must have nudged them to call me. I heard from Cindy Schmidler, Laurie Hall, Uncle Marc and Linda Two. It is wonderful to have the support of friends.

"One stress was relieved when my dad's surgery was a complete success. Praise the Lord! Another blessing was Grandma Bisson's acceptance of the Lord before she died. I had felt prodded by the Holy Spirit to go to her room one morning. My mom stayed with Alysa. We were by ourselves, and it was very quiet in her room. I put the side rails down on the bed and put my arms around my little grandma. Do you believe in God? Do you believe that Jesus died on the cross for your sins? He can come and live in your heart; all you have to do is ask him. Jesus loves you. I love you, too, and I want to see you in heaven. Will you accept him now?"

The dying lady took Linda's face between her hands and nodded her acceptance of the Lord, Jesus Christ. The family had been praying for 40 years that she would come to know the Lord and be saved. Linda was awed that God let her be the one to lead her on the path to eternal salvation. At her funeral two weeks later Dave sang "It Is Well with My Soul"

Linda concluded, "Don't ever give up praying for your loved ones."

It wasn't so well with Dave's soul, in Linda's opinion, when he took off for the golf outing at Boyne Mountain in Northern Michigan.

Linda: "It was one of those things. I wanted him home and felt that he should stay. He believed he needed a break and that he should go. After I arranged for a proficient, properly-trained aide to stay with Alysa at night, my pique with Dave dissolved. He did, indeed, need a break. When the aide refused money for her several nights' service, I thought she must have been an angel sent from heaven. Not all angels have wings and halos. They often show up as regular people who give of themselves to those in need."

CHAPTER NINE

On Friday, September 6, Dave strolled onto the first tee with dreams of eagles and birdies flying around in his head while Linda began her daily trip to see Alysa. She planned a limited routine of bathing and dressing Alysa.

"I had rolled Alysa over on her side so I could wash her back. She had her face buried in the pillow. I didn't think anything of it until I turned her back over. Her face and lips were blue! I alerted the nurse, who was preparing the linens for the bed."

"Liz! Alysa is turning blue."

"Oh, my god. She's so used to having the trache, she didn't realize she couldn't breathe pressed against the pillow," she said as she simultaneously pushed the panic or STAT button.

Both John and Pat from Respiratory ran into the room with Dr. Corbin in their wake. Linda was holding a tongue depressor in Alysa's mouth trying to keep her airway open. She quickly stepped aside as the breathing team approached.

"Here we go," John said as he inserted a plastic tube into Alysa's trachea to start the oxygen.

Dr. Corbin administered 4 mg of Ativan while Dr. Raines assessed Alysa's blood pressure and heart rate. "BP 142 over 87 and H.R. 197," he announced.

Alysa looked frightened. She stiffened, tensing her body and legs.

Linda spoke to the doctors, "What a way to start the day. Do you think her legs are stiff from a seizure or from being scared?"

"I don't think this was a seizure, but we'll order an EEG for verification," Dr. Corbin said.

Dr. Kent, the head neurologist, came to find Linda after the 4:00 EEG that afternoon. Linda reminded herself how much she appreciated the availability of the doctors.

He greeted mother and daughter then turned to Linda. "The EEG results are negative. This morning's episode wasn't a seizure. I thought you'd like to know."

"Oh, I'm so glad. Doctor, I'd like to ask you a few questions about seizures if you have the time."

"Sure. Shoot."

"Could you explain a seizure to me in layman's terms? And also, can you tell me how to differentiate between seizure activity and muscle spasms? Alysa is so physically active with her limb movements that I always wonder if it's a seizure."

"Okay. Let's begin Seizure 101. A seizure is caused by a spontaneous abnormal discharge of the neurons in the brain. The uncontrolled neuron activity causes signs and symptoms that vary according to the part of the brain that is malfunctioning. In short, whatever nerve cells are involved, a particular outcome is expected. A seizure is not a disease but a symptom of a central nervous system, or CNS, dysfunction. With me so far?"

"I think so. When Alysa had so many different behavioral responses at the onset of her illness, it meant that different parts of her brain were short-circuiting. All being caused by the infection, right?"

"Very good. A+ for you. Seizures can be caused by illness or injury to the brain, including infections, tumors, drug abuse, vascular lesions, and even birth deformities. There are two kinds of seizures: provoked and unprovoked. Provoked seizures are those brought on by high fevers, usually in children under five years, or those caused by metabolic or systemic disturbances. Those may be electrolyte imbalances, hypoglycemia, water intoxication, uremia, and CNS infections such as meningitis.

"Frequent recurrences of apparently unprovoked seizures are considered to be a seizure disorder or epilepsy. People with this form of seizure activity need anticonvulsant medication therapy."

"So, Alysa's seizures are the provoked kind?"

"That's right. Everyone has a seizure threshold—which can result in seizure activity. In your daughter's case, she contracted a virus and it passed through the blood/brain barrier. That is a filter around the Central Nervous System that exists to protect the brain from being invaded. Unfortunately, the infection slipped through her filter."

"That's why the spinal tap was so important," Linda said with resignation. "The one she didn't have in the first few days."

"Yes. An early identification of infection would have been most beneficial. Alysa has manifested both partial and generalized seizures referring to brain hemisphere involvement. In a simple partial seizure, there isn't always a loss of consciousness, but the part of the brain that is affected will produce symptoms. We have seen Alysa making repetitive motions and body movements. We call those automatisms. They are non-purposeful activity, such as her sticking her tongue out or waving her arms up and down. Usually there is confusion afterwards. A person with partial seizures is sometimes misunderstood and believed to require hospitalization for a psychiatric disorder," he concluded.

Linda just looked at the doctor. Finally she said, "Why didn't we have a doctor at the ER who would recognize these symptoms? Does the emergency room staff not know this kind of information? What went wrong?"

"It's a hard call. Usually EEG's or MRI's are needed to determine what's going on in the brain, especially when it's someone with an undiagnosed disorder. I'm afraid the ER staff just missed it."

"One last thing, Doctor. Back to my education. What about the clonic movements?"

"The actual term is myoclonic. It could be a seizure, too. It involves jerking of muscles, either focal—a localized infection, generalized or confined to the face."

"Great," Linda interrupted, "Alysa has both kinds."

"Yes, that's true. The first stage is called tonic—that's the rigid violent contraction of the muscle, which puts the limbs in a strained position. Then the second stage is the clonic phase, which involves rhythmic, bilateral contraction and relaxation of the extremities."

"You know, Doctor, even though I hate it that Alysa is going through this, it does give me some comfort to understand it and to demystify it. Her actions have technical and clinical explanations. I am very grateful for your taking the time to explain all of this to me. Now, if I can just remember it long enough to write it down for my derelict husband!"

Dr. Kent questioned Linda's comment with raised eyebrows. "Derelict?"

"Dave is on a golf vacation and I'm pouting."

The doctor grinned and said, "I'll be glad to talk to him, too. Besides, I'll want to hear all about his game. So long."

"Good-bye, Doctor, and thanks."

Ken spent his lunch hour with Alysa. Grandma Rivers split her time between the third, fourth and sixth floors. With her intuitive radar, Cindy called to see how Linda was holding up.

That evening, after a very tiring day for Alysa, the doctor from the St. Vincent's Rehabilitation facility came to assess her. His questions centered on Alysa's travels. Had she been out of the country? Up north in Michigan? Camping? Had she had a brain biopsy? The interview faltered. Alysa gave little indication of comprehension.

With Dave out of town, Linda Two ignored her doctor's cautioning of getting overtired and came to relieve Linda. "What kind of a day has it been?" she asked.

She got an earful. Finally, Linda kissed her daughter, prayed for her protection and left at 11:40 p.m. She was too tired to cry.

On Saturday, Grandpa Rivers had sneaked away from his surgical floor to check on his granddaughter. Imagine his surprise to see her standing! Ken and his father, Hank, had assisted Alysa in this newfound accomplishment and were worn out from the constant ups and downs.

"Hey, what's going on?" Andy asked.

Hank dramatically faked wiping his brow. "This girl's wearing us out!"

"That's all right with me," Ken said, "It's wonderful to have her out of that bed."

Andy chatted with the two other men and then turned to his granddaughter.

"Alysa, seeing you in that oversized T-shirt reminds me of

95

when you were a tiny thing and you helped me paint the living room. Remember? You were only four. You were so cute in that painter's cap that covered your entire head and the great big T-shirt that hung to the floor. I pulled the sofa out and I let you paint the entire wall. Remember? Then, I painted over it later when you weren't watching. You were so proud of that wall. 'That's my wall,' you told everyone."

He choked up a little as he finished his reminiscing.

Alysa's movements expanded on Sunday. Dave had returned, refreshed, from his golf outing. He treated Linda to a much-deserved dinner at Lelli's in Auburn Hills, and the couple rekindled their closeness with all recriminations forgotten. With Linda safely deposited at the Rivers', Dave returned to spend the night with Alysa. He slipped into the bathroom to brush his teeth, and when he reentered Alysa's room, he couldn't believe what he saw.

"Miss Houdini, what have you done to yourself?" he asked.

Somehow, Alysa had managed to position herself between the bed and the side bed rail with her knees touching the floor.

"Lys, you can't be comfortable. How in the world did you do that? Let me help get you back into the bed," Dave talked to his daughter as he tried to get her dislodged.

"Ugh. You're as unwieldy as 20 bags of potatoes. I can't reach the buzzer—guess I'll have to do this myself. Oh, and your Foley came out. Ouch. That had to hurt," he said as he finally managed to lift her.

Monday evening Pat, Pete, Christy and Becky Toth made one of their frequent visits.

"I'm glad you're here," Linda said. "Could you help me spread these blankets on the floor? And these pillows, too? Sometimes we like to give Lysa more moving room. Okay, Pete, can you get on her other side and grab her under her arm?"

Pete did as instructed and the two carefully laid Alysa down on the blankets.

"Linda, let's go for a walk," Pat suggested. "Pete and the girls will stay with Alysa awhile."

"Sounds good to me. Let's give Alysa some space," Linda said. "If you need anything, just push the call button for the nurse, okay?"

"Don't worry, we'll be fine. Christy and Becky can give Alysa all the news from church."

A mild no-sweater evening awaited the two friends. A walk in a park or on a wooded trail would have been preferable, but the parking lot perimeter would have to do. Pat and Linda shared their joys and frustrations of life on this earth and spoke with conviction of their future in eternity.

"How do people cope in this world if they don't know the Lord and don't know that he has prepared an eternal home?" Linda asked her friend. "If I didn't have that hope and promise, I don't know how I could endure this world."

Pat, an encourager and avid student of the scriptures agreed. "I think that is why there is so much discontent and desperation in the world today. People have forgotten that God made us to worship him and to live for him. Our purpose on earth is to learn all we can about the Father and to obey him. He wants us to have a relationship with him. He is a very real and personal God. 'For God so loved the world that he gave his one and only Son, that whoever believes in him shall not perish but have eternal life.'"

Discussing the Lord's prominence in their lives was a continuing source of strength to these two believers. The longer they strolled and talked, the more relaxed Linda became. Finally she regretfully acknowledged that it was time to go in.

They found Alysa sitting in the recliner chair.

Linda saw her and turned to Pete, "How did Alysa get into the chair? Pete, did you put her in it?"

Innocently, Pete replied, "No, she got into it herself."

Linda was incredulous. "She what?"

"Yeah, she sort of backwards crab-walked, or crawled, over to the chair and pulled herself up. I didn't know she couldn't do it."

"This is great progress, you guys. I'm so pleased," Linda said. Turning to Alysa she added, "Way to go, Lys. What are you going to be doing tomorrow? I can hardly wait to see."

The Toths gathered around Alysa and bowed their heads for prayer. Each family member thanked God for Alysa's accomplishments and gave him the credit. They prayed for her continued recovery and for her precious life. Alysa remained in the chair until 9:00 when the nurses readied her for bed.

Something new did occur within the next 24 hours, and Ken recorded it in the journal.

97

Wednesday, September 11
Day 122

12:00 Midnight. Alysa kissed me about ten times! Real ones! I haven't had one (kiss) in about three and a half months. No one could ever know how happy I am!!

During that day, Alysa showed remarkable improvement. She was alert, relaxed and even sat with her legs crossed. Such a normal gesture brought pangs to Linda's heart. Dr. Abraham visited while Alysa was sleeping, reporting the news that three rehab facilities had rejected Alysa. Her low-level status required too much medical attention.

Linda's reaction might have appeared strange to some. Linda: "Praise the Lord. I was not discouraged. I had prayed for the wrong doors to close. I wanted God to choose the right place for Alysa. I called Pat and Sandy Barnes to tell them of the outcome and to renew their prayers for the right facility for Alysa. When Pat said, 'Oh, no,' I reminded her of Psalms 33:11. 'That the plans of the Lord stand firm forever.'"

Incrementally, almost imperceptibly, progress occurred daily. On Sunday, September 15, Alysa was on her blanket retreat on the floor when she rolled from her tummy to a sitting up position. Nurse Terri was called to come in and see. Linda phoned Lisa, the Oakhill in-house social worker, who currently was searching for a suitable rehab for Alysa. She was thrilled. Alysa sat without losing her balance for 35 minutes. When she did lie down, she leaned on her elbows with her head in her hands and swung her legs, ankles crossed, in the air.

"Alysa looked like any teenager watching TV at a slumber party," said Linda.

"It was a sight for sore eyes," Dave added.

The room phone rang and Dave answered. It was Lisa.

Almost shouting, he relayed the news. "Linda, Lisa says that St. Vincent's Rehab has agreed to take Alysa! Praise the Lord!"

"Dave, let me talk to her, okay?" Linda took the phone and Dave hugged Alysa and conveyed the good news.

"Linda," said Lisa, "I dreamed that I had this very conversation with you and now it has happened. I'm just so glad there's a place for Alysa."

"We are so grateful for your help. When does she go?"

"She can be admitted on Wednesday. I'll fill you in on the procedure later. In the meantime, you will all have a chance to say your good-byes."

Dave's journal entry the night before moving day revealed his contemplative thoughts.

Tuesday, September 17
Day 128

11:00 a.m. As I sit here at the end of Alysa's bed and watch her beautiful smiling face, with her occasional yawns, I realize just how much progress our little girl has made. 129 days ago we were in the emergency room at Bellville Hospital. 128 days ago she was admitted and unfortunately misdiagnosed as to what her illness was. I still remember each night as if it were yesterday. I would pray, "Dear God, please make Alysa well. In Jesus' name." I don't know how many hundreds of times since then I have prayed that same prayer. I do know, however, that God is faithful and "as for me and my house, we will serve the Lord." Joshua 24:15. When we leave here Wednesday, September 18, Alysa's 129 days of hospitalization will end. Now that we are going to the Rehab Center it will be a new adventure and a new way to put our trust in God. Thank you, Jesus!

Interview with Dan Abraham

With kindness radiating from sensitive, brown eyes and with finely timbred, gentle words escaping his mouth, Dr. Dan Abraham might unwittingly confuse one of his patients or a patient's family member. Is this my doctor, they might wonder, or a Hollywood stand-in? His dark complexion coupled with curly black hair just touching the nape of his neck has most likely caused many a female head to turn and consider wanting to change Dan's eligible bachelor status. But Dan is not about appearances or looks. He is solely inflamed with being the best doctor that he can be. Fortunately for Alysa, he was her doctor.

Dan remembers his first encounter with Alysa:

It was late on a Friday night. I was on call at Oakhill Memorial. I got a phone call from an internal medicine resident whose opinion I knew I could trust. He told me of a young woman

I needed to see who was on the psychiatric floor although she had no prior history of psychological problems. She was seizing and was essentially unresponsive to her environment. The nurses had been watching her carefully, and they felt that something was really wrong.

I went in very early on Saturday morning and read the transfer charts that accompanied her from her former institution. It was clear to me that Alysa Conselyea was a very sick girl, one our neurological services needed to take very seriously. After I evaluated her, there was no doubt in my mind what I thought she had. I then spoke to the family to get a clearer picture, after which I called my boss to tell him he needed to come in. I explained the fevers, the seizures and how she presented elsewhere, at the former facility, and he agreed he needed to see her. To me, this was a key point: this girl, who never had seizures before, had no psychological history.

The parents, Linda and Dave, told me about the East Lansing hair show where Alysa thought something bad had happened. That entire scenario shouldn't have had any bearing on Alysa's treatment. It was important that a young girl, right in front of us, presented symptoms and from those a diagnosis could be made. In our minds, we never doubted the diagnosis the entire time. It was viral encephalitis, most likely herpes simplex. All the doctors at our hospital supported that diagnosis.

Alysa did not have an acute psychotic break. She had a mental status change. Her unusual behavior prior to her hospitalization, in my opinion, was caused by the infection. Toxic effect, changes in the blood, and even skin infections in the elderly can trip mental status changes. A brain infection can be slow or it can work fast. She showed symptoms for many days. Since the infection involves the temporal lobes, the area of dreamlike states, her worst nightmare of being physically or sexually harmed could have invaded her thought process. The Redken convention had a structured and supervised format, so I don't believe Alysa was attacked—except by a virus.

Very few viruses are so detrimental and damaging, but herpes simplex is the most common harmful virus. My boss ordered a lumbar puncture or spinal tap within five minutes of his arrival. The result was consistent with our diagnosis. Alys, my nickname for her, had a high white blood cell count and an elevated protein. It didn't tell us what it was for sure, but it didn't cancel our initial feelings or make us look elsewhere. Unfortunately, everything we did was after a time lapse of nearly two weeks from first onset of the illness. We had a strong suspicion of viral encephalitis but our testing could not pinpoint it. How did it get there? We don't know.

After the spinal tap we debated whether treatment would be of any benefit or were we too late. The treatment medications can have serious side effects. Opinions from the head of our internal medicine department and our infectious disease specialist, both outstanding physicians, gave us a green light. "Why the hell not?" was the reply from Dr. Kaye, the big boss. "We can take care of any side effect that will come up," he said. However, if you go only by book knowledge, it was truly too late. We chose to treat.

Alysa was getting excellent care on the psyche floor, but she was definitely not a psyche patient. The psychiatrists on the floor were not comfortable taking care of her medical illness, so she was moved to a medical floor. She had signs of tardive dyskinesia. Lip-smacking, oral movement, face and tongue manipulation—all side effects of anti-psychotic drugs, in particular, Haldol. These chorea-like movements eventually went away. I was glad. She could have had them for the rest of her life.

With Alysa I learned the subtleties of medicine. Day-to-day medicine, I call it. I would walk into her room and if she were sitting in a different way, I knew something was wrong. She received a great deal of medication because we were desperately trying to stop the brain seizures. Our only measurement of the seizing was by the EEG's. We ordered daily EEG's; they were always very bad. We planned a 24-hour EEG, but Alys tore off the wires after three hours. At least in that three-hour period we discovered she had some moments without the horrible seizing. Little consolation.

We sent samples of spinal fluid to the CDC in Atlanta and they requested more samples to send to alternate labs. They seemed to take special notice of our case and had a great interest that something unusual and frightening was happening to a young woman. We contacted most of the gurus in the field of neurology and infectious diseases. We searched the Internet and Physicians On-Line. There were no answers, no remedies, and no treatment. This very sick girl had a horrible hospital stay.

Except in one respect: every nurse, doctor, technician, maintenance and housekeeping person loved her. She never would have gotten off the ventilator if it hadn't been for the caring of the respiratory staff. They took a special interest in her and spent countless hours working with her—some on their own time because they felt she was so special. Many of the nurses felt vulnerable to see someone so ill who was near their own age. They were fearful of Alysa's final outcome.

What happened? they thought. This person is my age and all she did was wake up sick one morning. Did she bump into somebody on a bus somewhere and that person coughed in her face? Did she drink out of a cup that wasn't washed quite well enough? Some nurses were affected so deeply by Alysa's illness that they changed their careers. But most doted on Alysa and treated her like a sister.

Alys had complications. Pneumonia and responding poorly to medication were two of her nemeses. Dilantin and Tegretol, daily seizure meds, caused havoc. We constantly tried to figure out if her physical and mental improvements were caused by the medications or if she were getting better. Infection of the brain leaves scar tissue, which has its own ramifications. We continued to pursue other possibilities and other disease diagnoses with the hope that she wouldn't develop anything else.

While I treated Alysa, I never heard her say a word. Throughout her several month stay, Alys and her mother clearly communicated. It was similar to how a mother and her newborn baby interact. I would come into the room, stand and watch. Linda most often knew what Alys wanted. She could interpret Alys' discomfort by a look on her face. She looked into Alys' eyes and talked to her. We'd try to figure out for hours why Alysa writhed in bed. Mom would walk in, take one look, grab a pillow from the other bed and put it under Alys' head—solution found.

The official terminology for Alys' state is "not responsive to her environment." She did not have appropriate reactions. She could not protect herself. She would see you but look right through you. At times she was heavily sedated, medically induced. Although I would not label her comatose or catatonic, medically speaking, a lay person would consider her to be in a coma. She sometimes responded to her mother and she would jerk away if pinched or prodded. She definitely was encephalopathic, or confused.

I personally got to know Linda and Dave very well. After the first time I met them, it was impossible not to do everything I could for their daughter. They are an amazing couple. They faced hard times and difficult events, but it only seemed to make them stronger. I think only one in a hundred couples could endure what they did and survive. That kind of desire and dedication from family members is rare. They knew they had to be there twenty-four hours a day in order to get the best care for Alys. And they did it.

All of the doctors wanted to help the Conselyeas with their daughter. We just wanted to wrap this little girl up in a blanket and send her home as fast as we possibly could. But it seemed like that was never going to happen. The Conselyeas had their faith. But I questioned if there is a God or not. Alysa didn't deserve being sick and put into such dreadful situations. I'm waiting for the answer if God exists.

Ken, Alysa's boyfriend, overwhelmed me by his devotion to her. If this match weren't made in heaven, then there is nothing out there worthwhile if this doesn't work. I don't think I could bear the things he had to stomach. Decision-wise, he had no say. He had to just stand by and accept everything.

I wondered if he was waiting for permission to walk away. Being single, I thought I understood. I took him aside and mentioned that he could walk away and no one would blame him or think poorly of him. He understood he could walk—but he had the courage and the conviction to stay. He is one great guy from another great family.

I became obsessive and compulsive regarding her care. Away on a medical conference, I called in at least three times a day. Unfavorable things seemed to happen when I was gone. Calling in was my preventative method. I awoke at 4:00 one morning, feeling that something had happened, and called the night nurse. She got angry with me, but I hated being out of the loop. If anyone gave Alys a Tylenol, I wanted to know why. I didn't want any little thing to be overlooked, because then it was two steps back when we were measuring progress in inches.

My training through Dr. Owens emphasized that doctors practiced medicine for the patients. Ego, money, status, and hospital policy had no influence. We were taught to treat all patients whether they have insurance or not, to do everything possible, no matter what the medical condition, and to care for the patient.

This philosophy was not typical at all facilities. If a patient couldn't pay for an MRI, we did it anyway if that was what was needed. Our administration never came to us to even hint that we discharge Alysa although the care she was receiving could be done at a nursing home. There was never a thought to take away the room where Dave and Ken stayed. It never came up. She was a difficult patient to make better, but our philosophy was to stick with her as long as it took—even if it took two years to remove her from the vent.

If we had known what she faced when she left us to go to St. Vincent's, we wouldn't have let her go. We would have loved to have her back. I stayed in close contact with the family as I held on to what the most senior guru of neurology said to me when I asked if she were going to get better. He has the uncanny ability to walk into a room and know the diagnosis without even shaking the patient's hand. With confidence and knowing, his response was spoken with words as smooth as silk, "Yes, she'll get better."

CHAPTER TEN

A steady stream of well-wishers paraded through room 416 on Wednesday: Dr. Kent, Dr. Corbin, Dr. Raines, Dr. Rice, Pat and Karen from Respiratory, Aunt Carol, Ken, Joe, the security guard, Dr. Abraham, Joan from housekeeping who brought Alysa a Bill Gaither tape, Grandma and Grandpa Rivers, Linda Two and of course the proud parents.

Lisa explained the dismissal and admittance arrangements to Dave amid the poignant farewells. Dr. Raines, wearing an electric-blue sports jacket, approached Alysa.

He knelt down beside the bed and took Alysa's right hand in his. "When you get well, I'm going to take you out for dinner and dancing—on me! That's a promise."

Alysa put her arms around the kind-hearted doctor, hugged him tightly and said, "Good-bye."

The expected wheelchair escort arrived and Alysa was maneuvered into it. With her personal gear packed, mementos, tape player, tapes and stuffed animals crammed into a cardboard box, the Conselyea entourage left the room. As Alysa was wheeled into the hallway, the nurses had gathered for her departure, most shedding tears unabashedly. To everyone's great astonishment, Alysa stood up from the wheelchair and carefully, placing one foot in front of the other, slowly walked the length of the nurse's station. All felt they were witnessing a miracle. Smiles burst out on faces with accolades of "Way to go, Alysa," "Yea! Alysa," "Praise the Lord," "Good-bye," "God bless," and from Linda, "God is so good."

A small caravan headed for St. Vincent's Rehab on the northeast side of Detroit. A tailgate party was planned to welcome Alysa to her new home.

Linda: "This time the ride in the ambulance was one of joy. I felt exhilarated that my daughter was out of the hospital and was going to begin her physical recovery. I told Alysa what to expect.

"Honey, you are going to love this place. Your dad and I came over yesterday to look around. You will be in a semi-private room just for the day, and then you'll have your own private room for your entire stay. Isn't that wonderful?"

Alysa probably heard and understood what her mother was telling her, but her vision was focused outside on the passing landscape, and she did not respond.

Once in the parking lot, Grandpa Rivers, Linda Two, Linda and Dave all welcomed Alysa. There was no food at this particular tailgate affair—just hugs, kisses, hopes and prayers for Alysa's new adventure. Andy and Linda Two waved good-bye and threw kisses as Alysa was wheeled away.

Alysa met her new nurse, Leann, who ordered a custom fitted wheelchair with a high-backed head support. In just minutes the personalized wheelchair arrived.

"Could we take Alysa outside and give her a tour of the grounds?" Dave asked.

"Sure, go right ahead. I'll get her chart started," Leann said.

The family exited through the automatic sliding doors into the mid-morning sunshine. They headed for a path with trees where some still-blooming flowers dotted the landscape. A few benches and a table stood near a small pond with a bubbling water fountain.

"This is a great place, Lys. Don't you just love it?" said her dad. Alysa processed her new location without acknowledgment.

A young woman walked over to them. "Oh, here you are. I'm Rachel, one of Alysa's aides. I thought I'd get her blood pressure and temp while you're out here."

"Just like at the hospital, huh Lys? Yeah, right."

Dave and Linda couldn't help feeling upbeat even though they had some anxiety at the thought of again dealing with doctors and nurses unfamiliar with this difficult case.

"I think we should pray before we go back in," Dave suggested. They bowed their heads and took their praises and concerns to their God.

"Dear Father," Dave prayed quietly. "You are the awesome God, the Creator of this world. We thank you and praise you for your mighty works with our precious daughter. Lord, you have continued to answer our prayers, and we have the promise that you will never forsake us. As we are about to start a new phase of Alysa's care, we just ask that you give her strength and healing. We thank you for the doctors and nurses who will care for her. We know that your timing is not always ours, but we trust that you will make Alysa well. Watch over her and protect her. In Jesus' name, we pray. Amen." They hesitated a few seconds and headed confidently into the unforeseen.

They navigated the hallway to Alysa's temporary room. Alysa wasn't doing very well. Her eyes focused off to one side and blinked continuously. The speech therapist came in and introduced herself. Linda mentioned that Alysa was two hours late in getting her Phenobarbital. Nurse Jenni checked the roster to get a sitter for the night so Linda and Dave could get a good night's sleep—together.

"Sounds good to me," he whispered to Linda with an attempt at a leer.

She shushed him, but with a tolerant grin.

Jenni said, "Good news. I've got someone lined up to stay the night. Now, we'll get Alysa ready for a shower."

"A shower?" Dave repeated. "This is her first shower in four months. I love this place!"

Ken arrived after work to see a shiny clean and happy Alysa. "How's my girl?" he asked while he leaned down for a kiss. "Have you had any dinner?" he asked the Conselyeas.

"Not yet. I don't know if we can eat here on short notice or not. I'll go find out," Linda said. Dave and Ken chatted about the new surroundings until Linda returned.

"The rule generally is that they want four hours' advance notice if we want a meal. They would make an exception tonight. The menu is meat loaf and mashed potatoes. What do you think?"

"There's a McDonald's, a Bill Knapps and a Coney Island a

few blocks away," Ken informed them.

"Why don't I go and pick up something," Dave suggested. I hate for us all to leave her right now. What do you guys want?"

"Anything but McDonald's," Linda said.

"Anything's fine with me," Ken said, and gave Dave directions to the restaurants.

"I'll surprise you," he said, fishing for the car keys in his coat pocket.

Dave returned with their old standby of fried chicken and its fixings from Chicken Shack. They picnicked in Alysa's room and wished she could share in their meal. She was getting thinner while they were all adding weight from 129 days of their fast food, grab-a-bite regime. Linda and Dave left at 10:00 p.m. and Ken left at 11:00, after the sitter had arrived. The day rated high on their scale.

Two of the facility's doctors examined Alysa first thing Thursday morning. Dr. Kinneman, the head doctor for the rehab center, and Dr. Amani, Alysa's internist, privately compared their assessments. Then she was off to physical therapy. Alysa had the luxury of having the therapist and the room all to herself—no distractions. Most of the myriad of equipment available suited the more advanced patients. For Alysa, her legs and ankles were massaged, extended and flexed accordingly. Next came sitting and standing.

"She's doing very well," Darleen, the therapist, told Linda.

They did some arm movements, too. The total workout lasted 30 minutes before Alysa seemed to tire.

Back in the room the speech therapy started. Alysa's tongue was swabbed with a lemon flavor to stimulate her taste buds. Relearning how to swallow was practiced with sips of grape juice from a spoon. Alysa responded well to the instructions she received all morning.

Once the word of Alysa's medical journey circulated the facility, nurses and workers stopped in to share personal stories of their friends or loved ones. The occupational therapist was one of the first to come in.

"I just wanted you to know that my sister had viral encephalitis, too. She was with her boyfriend riding in his car when she had her first seizure. When she first went to the hospital, she was diagnosed as a psychiatric case. It's a long story. But, I thought you would have some comfort in knowing that she has completely recovered."

"Thanks for telling me. I'm so glad for your sister and all of your family. We believe that God is going to heal Alysa, too," Linda said.

A nurse volunteered her own personal history to Linda. "Eight years ago I had a traumatic head injury. The doctors gave up on me and told my husband that I would be a vegetable. By God's grace I recovered. Because of my experience I decided to go to nursing school. I failed my first three classes, but I didn't give up. I persevered and with God's help, I graduated. And here I am," she finished.

Encouraged by her words, Linda said, "It is so good to hear positive outcomes of tragic situations. Frowns and dire forecasts don't belong in a sick room. Do you know the Lord?"

"Yes, I'm a believer. God is my rock and my salvation."

They talked awhile on the subject that always delighted sisters of the faith, their Jesus.

Friends came to visit Alysa and took her outside. A passing truck made horrific noises and Alysa became very upset. She covered her ears and refused to remove her hands as long as she remained outside. Consequent trips outside elicited the same behavior.

Alysa's case was scheduled for staff review at noon on Friday. Because she was admitted on a week's trial basis, Alysa's staying in the rehab depended on her performance. Alysa had slept soundly the night before and had slept all morning. Darleen came in and sat and stroked Alysa, running her fingers through her hair. Still, she didn't wake up.

"I'll come back this afternoon," she said.

John and Cindy had been in town and came to visit before they had to catch their plane to Indy. Cindy talked to Alysa.

"We got a new puppy, Alysa. Know what we named him? Nestle. Can you guess what color he is? Yeah, he's brown. Adam just loves him. You'd like him, too. Remember, now, you have to try hard to get better. You have to give 110%. Okay? I know you can do it," Cindy said, winding down her pep talk.

Linda was having difficulty concentrating on her friends during their short visit. She noticed that Alysa was biting her tongue and that her eyes were darting all around the room. A sinking feeling overwhelmed her. Oh, no, not again, she thought. Something was wrong.

At 2:00 Darleen returned. "We'll just do the therapy here in the room today," she said.

But Alysa was non-responsive. She was lethargic—like a wet noodle.

"I think we'll get Jenni in here to check her, okay?"

Jenni assessed Alysa and called for someone in neurology. Dr. Stephanie Baskin made the diagnosis. "She is definitely having partial seizures. We'll change some of her medications and wait for results."

That evening when Dave arrived from work, he found Linda in the parking lot, crying.

"Sweetheart, what's wrong? What happened? Do you want to go in?"

"No, let's just stay out here," she said between sniffles. "Lysa definitely had seizure activity today. She didn't respond to therapy and she was out of it."

Touching her elbow and guiding her away from the public parking lot, Dave said, "Let's walk around the courtyard, want to?"

"Okay. I just don't understand. It seems like we take one step forward and then two steps backwards. I had such high hopes for Lysa here."

"Now, don't get discouraged. Don't give up. Have faith. Remember God's promise to you. God wouldn't have brought Lysa here to leave us stranded. We just have to trust and obey him."

"I know you're right, but I can't separate my emotions from what I know he will do. It's so hard."

Dave continued to console his wife. As so often happens in stressful and traumatic events, a couple's individual strengths wax and wane. This seesaw response is predictable. When one is weak, the other is strong. When one is up, the other is down.

Holding her closely, he asked, "Ready to go back in?"

"I'd rather stay here like this," she said, snuggling in his embrace.

"Can't get enough of me, is that it?"

"Yeah, something like that." His humor had broken the tense time, and with arms around each other, they prepared to face the next hurdle.

"Mom called and said that Marc's flying in tomorrow. I hope Alysa is better and that she recognizes him. He'll be so disappointed if she doesn't."

"When does his flight arrive? Do you want me to pick him up?"

"No, Dad is going to get him. His arrival time is 3:30 but with weather and traffic delays, who knows when he'll actually get in."

* * * * *

Marc carefully threaded his way through the crowded jetway, anxious to see his dad and his family. He spotted the tall frame of Andy Rivers and yoo-hooed in his direction.

"Hi, ya, Pop. How are you? You look great."

"What did you expect—that I'd be an old man just because of a little surgery? The docs did a good job."

They fell in line behind the throngs, "Have you got any checked baggage?"

"Nope. Traveling light. So how is everybody?"

"Well, I'm afraid I've got some bad news."

"What? Alysa?"

Their pace slowed as they funneled onto the moving sidewalk. They stepped to the right so those in a hurry could pass by them and they could continue their conversation.

"You won't get to see Alysa in rehab. She's been admitted back into the hospital. This time she is in St. Vincent's Hospital, the main facility for St. Vincent's Rehab."

"What happened?" Marc asked, shaking his head.

"She's having constant seizures again and the staff felt she needed more medical attention than she could receive at rehab. It's a darn shame. We thought she was really getting better."

The favorite uncle and the adored grandfather pushed through the terminal doors in silence, each deep in his own thoughts about the young girl they loved so very much.

CHAPTER ELEVEN

On that 132nd day since Alysa's initial hospitalization, Dave had arrived at the rehab center at 6:30 a.m. He was so tired that he planned to relieve the night sitter after a quick last minute snooze in the car. A nurse tapped on his window.

Waking with a start, Dave muttered, "Uh, what? What time is it?" Then he recognized Leann.

"Good morning, Mr. Conselyea. Well, it's 10:30…."

"Ten-thirty? It can't be. Oh, I'm so sorry, I should have come in hours ago."

"That's all right. Mrs. Conselyea called and was concerned, so I'm the search party."

Gathering his belongings, Dave bounded out of the car and headed to the entrance with the nurse.

"So, how is Alysa this morning? Is she any better?" he asked with undisguised hope as he opened the door for the nurse. Once alongside in the hallway she informed him.

"I'm afraid not. We administered Ativan last night because of her seizure activity. The doctors want to move her to our main hospital in Detroit. She'll be leaving this afternoon for St. Vincent's at 6 Mile and Mack Avenue."

"Boy, am I sorry to hear that. We really like this place. Poor Alysa."

That last thought contrasted to the Alysa Dave saw when he

walked into her room. She had been given a shower and shampoo, sleeping through both, and she looked so pretty and peaceful lying in her bed. He called Linda and gave her the news. Linda, in turn, called her prayer warriors and the church, seeking spiritual support.

St. Vincent's Hospital, home number four for Alysa, was a huge complex. It made the other two hospitals seem like clinics in comparison. Dr. Baskin, the neurologist who had seen Alysa at the rehab, was still in charge of her care. She ordered an EEG and, upon reading the results, explained her intent to the parents.

"We're transferring your daughter to the MICU, or Medical Intensive Care Unit. We want to initiate a deep coma so her brain can completely rest. To do that, we will administer a Pentobarbital drip. After two or three days, we will slowly decrease the drip and check her brain activity," she explained.

Dave asked, "Is this a normal procedure—one that's done all the time?"

Choosing her words carefully, Dr. Baskin said, "It is not a rare treatment, but it is done only when we have a patient with severe provoked seizures—like Alysa's. I think it is time to do something aggressive instead of reacting to each seizure episode. We will keep her sedated until the seizure activity comes to a complete stop."

Guided by the doctor, they stepped into a Star Trek environment. The gleaming machines, odd contraptions, multiple dials and hoses, supply-stacked carts and other-worldly high tech gear of the MICU overwhelmed them. Unaware of their gawking, Dr. Baskin continued, "Here, I'll introduce you to the MICU doctor and Alysa's nurse. This is Matt, the head MICU nurse, and this is Dr. Ormond."

The automatic handshakes and hellos masked the shell-shock that Linda and Dave were experiencing. The Conselyeas huddled outside the MICU with Linda Two and Grandma Rivers and discussed and digested this new tactic. They overstayed the allowed visiting hours. Reluctantly, at 10:00 they prepared to leave.

Linda went to her sleeping daughter's side and with her eyes watering, she softly prayed, "Dear Lord, please guard and protect Alysa tonight and let her feel your presence all around her. Protect her thoughts and dreams. Thank you for bringing us to this facility. May your will be done. In Jesus' name, Amen."

Matt spoke reassuringly to the parents as they were leaving, "I will watch Alysa very closely tonight. Don't you worry about her for a minute. I won't leave her side. She's my only patient. We'll be putting her back on the respirator, and several computers'll monitor her as well. She'll be fine," he said. Leaving her in capable hands, both seen and unseen, they left.

After three days, the EEG's continued to show seizure activity, even with the Pentobarbital drip. The drip was increased. Additional anti-seizure medication, Lamictol, a drug just-approved by the FDA, was given. An MRI was the next diagnostic procedure ordered. A lumbar puncture had shown no irregularities.

Linda: "We weren't allowed to be with Alysa for EEG's or MRI's, so the hospital chapel became my retreat. The room whispered peace and the muted coloring surrounded me with comfort. The altar had a beautiful rough-hewn cross. Behind it a back-lit stained glass panel depicting Christ as the Shepherd shone brightly. I got on my knees and prayed to my Shepherd, knowing his flock was praying from their homes, offices and cars around the community and the country. I repeated one of my favorite verses, Philippians 4:67, 'Do not be anxious about anything, but in everything, by prayer and petition, with thanksgiving, present your requests to God. And the peace of God, which transcends all understanding, will guard your hearts and minds in Christ Jesus.'"

Marc had been in several times to see his niece. He would hold her hand and try to keep from crying.

"I don't know how you can stand all of this," he said, with a sweep of his hand around the machine-filled cubicle. "God has got to hear our prayers and heal her."

"He will in his timing," Linda answered. "We can't just demand things to fit our desires and our schedule. We have to trust God that his timing is perfect," she said to her brother.

"How can you accept that, Linda? Where do you get that kind of faith?"

"There will be a time, in eternity, that everything on earth will make sense to us. There is a greater picture that we aren't allowed to see. To ask for that knowledge now is the same thing Adam and Eve did when they ate the fruit from the tree. They knew God, but

Satan tricked them into wanting to be God. Satan is alive and well and working in our world. He casts doubts and distracts us from our main purpose in life: to honor, obey and trust the Lord. I will not let Satan get a toe in the door. I will trust God's will for Alysa's life. God told me he would heal Alysa and I hold on to that promise."

"You're an amazing woman, Sis. You really are."

"No, it is God who is amazing."

*   *   *   *   *

With all the medications bombarding her body and with her inactivity, Alysa developed secondary and tertiary conditions.Her immune system was depleted so she contracted pneumonia. A rash erupted on her tongue, called thrush. She became swollen and bloated and had a bowel blockage. She was running a fever. Add to that the EEG glue that had to be scrubbed out of her hair each day and the result was one sorry, pathetic-looking patient.

Pastor Jim visited and brought words of encouragement to Dave and Linda. His casual, unhurried visit was directed solely to the needs of those in the room—as if he didn't have 17 other people to visit that day.

"Linda, you've been so good about calling the church to ask for prayer. And people always want an update. So we have dedicated a corner in the Sunday bulletin as 'Alysa's Corner.' We want you to call the church office every Thursday and tell us the exact needs that Alysa has so everyone can pray specifically. Mention the prayers that have been answered, too. Could you do that?"

Overcome with gratitude, Linda replied, "That is so kind. The prayers mean so much to all of us. I'll certainly call on Thursdays. Dave, you remind me, okay?

"What the church did for Ken and his family was so very thoughtful. I know Linda Beaudoin plans to send a letter, but she told me that they were overwhelmed with the food, staples and other products. She didn't understand how people who didn't even know her could give so freely. With her Lupus diagnosis and with Ken paying all the bills, it was a hard time."

"That's what the church is all about," Pastor Jim replied. "When someone is having financial trouble, those who care and want to show the love of Christ are compelled to help. They wanted to help Ken and his mother because they knew how much help they were to you. I'll pass along the thanks."

Warming up to the subject, Linda asked, "Jim, you know that little café on Dixie and Andersonsville Road, L.A. Café?"

Jim nodded.

"Well, Alysa worked there for six months or so and the owner, Heidi, visited a few weeks ago when Alysa was at Oakhill. She said that she and her husband Darren wanted to help. They offered to organize a fund raiser to collect donations for Alysa's medical bills and care. They wanted to do something tangible. Knowing that people genuinely care about Alysa is so encouraging. We declined their sincere offer, but isn't that wonderful?"

"We have a wonderful God."

Linda recalled yet another instance of people unknown to them lifting their hearts in prayer. "Oh, and there was a nurse at Oakhill, a black woman, who would come into Alysa's room and pray with all her heart and soul. I've never heard anyone pray so passionately. She told me that her entire church was praying for Alysa. And they don't know her either. Alysa got to meet the nurse just before we left there."

After Jim's departure, renewed and thankful hearts remained.

Sunday, September 29
Day 140

6:30 a.m. Good Morning, Girlfriend! Your number one boyfriend is here. Looks pretty good (but not very comfortable). H.R.=86, Blood Ox=99, BP=103/57 (75 maybe?). Temp has been good. 7:05 a.m. Dr. Tom Berto stopped in. Very knowledgeable. Asked if I understood her condition. I had him explain it. Her seizures are called "non-convulsive status," which means they don't show any outward signs and are pretty much constant. This happens when the brain is allowed to operate unchecked, and the person can't stop it due to brain scarring and over-exertion. Since she can't control the seizure on her own, they use drugs (Pentobarb) to do it. The goal is to let her brain rest and cool down enough so that she can regain control. Even when the seizures are under control, there is always a possibility of them re-occurring. Sometimes it takes a day for the brain to rest enough, sometimes three days, sometimes a week. They've tried resting one day a few times, and it hasn't worked. He said yesterday they had a lot of trouble controlling them. He isn't going to touch the Pentobarb today. They will try tomorrow (Monday) and if that doesn't work, they may keep her under for as long as three days to a week. The problem with that is that the body isn't made to just sit there, so complications increase: blood, lung, urinary infections and bed sores. He said the infectious disease people didn't think the infections were serious, so far. He said that there is no drug to heal the brain. All they can do is let it rest and give it time to heal itself. How long it takes for that to happen they don't know. He said that the non-convulsive status seizures are very rare. They might see two to three cases a year. Hopefully I asked the right questions. I wish Linda and Dave could have talked to him! I also asked about the MRI. He said there was nothing unusual. He asked what the other doctors said about the previous lesions they found. I said not much. He said it probably had very little to do with her problem. So, it sounds like this MRI showed nothing. He said that they usually aren't very useful in these cases.

12:00 Linda Two here. EEG still showed seizures so they are putting her back on Pentobarb and will do another about 1:00 p.m. today.

1:30 p.m. Linda, Dad and Ken here. Lo and behold, but who is in the room but good old Dr. Abraham. Also Carolyn Mack and her kids came to see Alysa. They kicked us out at 2:00 to finish a second EEG. At 2:30 we said good-bye to Dr. A and came back in. H.R.= 85, Blood Ox=99, and B.P. 103/57.

While Alysa was in the induced coma, her family continued speaking to her and reading books and scripture. The dialect in *Cold Sassy Tree* by Olive Ann Burns took a well-tuned tongue.

I knew he was real excited because he kept scratching his head fast. But he didn't act like I'd been snatched from hell or go on about a maggotty horse hoof on the railroad tracks or how I had to pray to God to use the life He had so mercifully spared. Grandpa reached across the table and put his hand on my arm, just for a second, then poked me in the ribs and said, "By George, gittin' ran over by a train must a-been some experience!" He acted like it was something to remember instead of something to forget. With the

117

way he took it so casual, and the relief of getting it told, I felt like I'd been stuck back together. But one thing worried me. "Grandpa, you think I'm alive cause it was God's will?"

"Naw, you livin' cause you had the good sense to fall down 'twixt them tracks."

"Maybe God gave me the idea."

"You can believe thet, son, if'n you think it was God's idea for you to be on thet there trestle in the first place. What God give you was a brain. Hit's His will for you to use it—p'tickler when a train's comin'."

Resting my chin in my hand, I thought about that while Grandpa finished up his pie. I felt awful tired. "Sir, do you think it was God's will for Bluford Jackson to get lockjaw and die?"

Grandpa spoke kindly. "The Lord don't make firecrackers, son. Hit's jest too bad pore Blu didn't be more careful when he was shootin'm off."

"You don't think God wills any of the things that happen to us?"

"Maybe. Maybe not. Who knows?"

"Mama and Papa think He does."

Grandpa licked some meringue off his fork while he pondered. Finally he said, "Life bullies us, son, but God don't. He had good reasons for fixin' it where if'n you git too sick or too hurt to live…."

"Excuse me, Mrs. Conselyea, I need to talk to you about Alysa's reactions to certain drugs. I'm sorry to interrupt," Dr. Baskin apologized.

"That's okay," said Linda putting the bookmark between the pages. "I've got the list of the drugs she has reacted to right here in our journal," she said, flipping its pages. She read them off, "Dilantin, Amphotericin, Vancomycin, Haldol, and all sulfa drugs."

"That's quite a long list. Are you sure she is allergic to Dilantin?"

"Yes, I'm positive. She had fevers after it was administered."

"Well, I'd like to give her Dilantin," the doctor concluded, not seeming to trust Linda's judgment.

The Pentobarbital drip had its own consequences. The side effects Alysa suffered from it included drowsiness, lethargy, hangover, nausea, vomiting, rash, somnolence, agitation, confusion, hypotension (low blood pressure), constipation and headache. Adverse reactions stacked up like so many discards in the game of Canasta. Her face broke out with a case of acne that would shock a dermatologist. The culprits? Two new drugs: Tegretol and Phentobarbitol.

At this point in their medical voyage, a woman from Faith Baptist appeared with a conviction that the Holy Spirit touched her heart to visit Alysa and to read scripture to her. Laneen Manchester had tried to sign up on the prayer sheet at church and found that all the time slots were taken. That was her indication that she was to visit in person. The Conselyeas were touched by her desire to minister to them and to Alysa. Her vigor was matched by her endurance as she tirelessly read Psalm after Psalm.

Friday, October 4, was the new projected day to stop the Pentobarb drip. Friends doubled their prayers and support for Linda and Dave. Laurie Hall came early to pray, sing and read to Alysa. Alysa's eyes were open, but they were doll's eyes. Undaunted, Laurie read the twenty-fourth Psalm.

"The earth is the Lord's and everything in it, the world, and all who live in it; for he founded it upon the sea and established it upon the waters. Who may ascend the hill of the Lord? Who may stand in his holy place? He who has clean hands and a pure heart, who does not lift up his soul to an idol or swear by what is false. He will receive blessing from the Lord and vindication from God his Savior…."

"I'm afraid I'm going to have to ask you ladies to leave now. It's time for Alysa's bath," the nurse informed Linda and Laurie. "Then she'll be getting the EEG. You can come back at 5:00."

"Just let us say a prayer and we'll be gone," Linda requested.

Laurie prayed for Alysa the prayer that they were all saying, "Lord, God, we ask that you take these seizures away from Alysa. Heal her, protect her and watch over her." The prayer partners took the elevator down to the chapel to expand on their petitions to El Elyon, the Most High God.

While they were in the chapel, Alysa's temperature shot up to 104.5. The nurse gave her a cooling bath to bring it back down. An hour later, Linda and Lorrie left the chapel. With renewed resolve they were ready to face whatever God had in store.

They got the results of the EEG from the nurse. "Dr. Baskin says there is no status epilepticus, but there is slight brain activity. We are observing Alysa for 12 hours and we are to notify the doctor immediately if there is any head movement. She is off the drip."

With elated heart, Lorrie said, "I'll call the prayer chains and Sandy and Pat and get the requests rolling. Call me as soon as you know anything."

Linda hugged her friend and said, "Thanks for everything. You are an answer to my prayers."

At 9:30 the next morning, Alysa had an upper body seizure. She was put back on the Pentobarbital drip.

Interview with Sandy Barnes

With dark curls bobbing and intense blue eyes shining, Sandy Barnes commands her listener's attention. This petite lady with her heart-shaped face cuts a surprisingly imposing figure as she delivers her Bible Study Fellowship lectures. The passion of the subject matter gives Sandy her stature. The vibrant relationship that she has with Christ is what she hopes for every BSF member.

Sandy tells her story:

My family didn't attend church, but I always loved going to Vacation Bible School. My mother would sometimes take us to three different sessions in one summer. Even as a youngster, I knew I needed a Savior. I had a keen awareness of God. And besides, I was afraid of the consequences: going to hell. I accepted Christ at one of those sessions and had security in that action, but my acceptance was superficial. I remember praying when I was in need. At thirty-something and with children, my husband Brent and I made Christ the Lord of our lives.

Realizing that my own introduction to Jesus and salvation began at a tender age, I value children's teachers and leaders who teach about Christ. Never underestimate what children's workers contribute to God's kingdom.

Linda Conselyea came to the Clarkston BSF on the invitation

120

of a friend. She demonstrated her responsiveness to the word of God. She showed willingness to apply what she learned. I could see her grow spiritually one week to the next.

Later, eager to give of herself, she became one of those special children's leaders. She taught the children of those who attended the lecture and small group sessions. Bible Study Fellowship exists to train Christian leaders to participate in their own churches and communities. Knowing and applying scripture enables the believer to establish a relationship with Jesus Christ. Those who are called to leadership positions commit themselves without reservation to the cause of Christ. Linda embraces commitment.

We scheduled BSF leadership meetings each week on Mondays before our large session on Tuesdays. We socialized, planned and shared prayer requests within our leadership group and spent time getting to know each other better. We had 45 or 50 leaders involved when Alysa got sick.

I vividly remember trying to reach Linda on a Wednesday before my son's wedding. She had promised me a recipe I could use at the rehearsal dinner Thursday night. She finally called me very late on Wednesday night. Along with the recipe ingredients, she listed the strange symptoms that her daughter exhibited. The confusing account left me wondering if Alysa's problems were physiological, psychological or spiritual. Nevertheless, I acknowledged Linda's request for prayer and passed it on. Our leaders continued our prayer support for the many months of Alysa's illness.

Our nine-month Bible study ended in May so leaders' meetings stopped, too. As the seriousness of Alysa's problems mounted, we kept the leaders apprised so we could pray for the medical staff, for guardianship, for healing, for understanding and for whatever urgent need arose. Connecting with Linda became impossible as she practically lived at the hospital. Brenda Cox and Lorrie Hall, both BFS leaders, became our contact people for information.

My first visit to the hospital resulted in shock. I had not imagined the extent of the situation. Alysa, unable to sit, with eyes staring blankly, appeared to be in a catatonic state. Yet the room was filled with an amazing peace. Linda's demeanor enveloped the room. Her calmness, tender speech and caring for Alysa and for everyone else impressed me. She spoke to Alysa as if she were cognizant. She interpreted Alysa's minimal body language and did not become frustrated with Alysa's inability to communicate. She had phenomenal patience.

Her constant faith never wavered. Quite honestly, I doubted Alysa's chances for recovery, although I never voiced it to Linda. She prayed with confidence and supported her prayers with scripture.

If she experienced temptation to doubt, it never showed. In her requested prayers for her daughter she expected complete restoration. Her prayers mirrored the directions given in Matthew. "But when you pray, go into your room, close the door and pray to your Father who is unseen. Then your Father, who sees what is done in secret, will reward you. And when you pray, do not keep babbling like pagans, for they think they will be heard because of their many words. Do not be like them, for your Father knows what you need before you ask him."

Because of Linda's example, so many others have grown in their faith. She depended fully on the Lord. God gave her an opportunity and she chose to use it for good. When trials and heartbreak come into our lives, we can use them for God's glory or we can waste these opportunities. Linda used them. Her commitment to God did not depend on her circumstances. That is one of the lessons I have learned.

God has told us in his word that he wants us to love him more than anything else—including our children. When our child is affected, we often blame God and direct anger at him. Our love for him does not depend on what he does with our loved ones.

I remember a conversation I had with Linda. She never questioned how the Lord could do this to her only child. In fact, Linda told me she had prayed fervently that her dad would come back to the Lord. She told God "Whatever it takes—even if it means losing my only daughter."

We received the blessing by witnessing her steadfastness. The bleakest situation imaginable can be used to glorify God. No matter what happened to Alysa, Linda loved God. He honored her by giving her complete fulfillment and joy.

To this day she chooses to be a giver, not a receiver. Whenever we assist others, it helps us through our own trials. I learned that from Linda.

Interview with Brenda Cox

Neat, meticulous, perfectly manicured, great complexion—"together"—all describe Brenda Cox. It's hard to believe she's a grandmother eight times over. Her love of people is a badge that shines for all to see. She is one of those people that you like immediately. That's probably why Brenda and Linda were drawn to each other.

Brenda tells how Linda and she became friends:

I met Linda at a women's retreat at Camp Co-Beac. I remember being particularly impressed with Linda's openness and her caring personality. Later, one Sunday in 1988, Dave, Linda and Alysa came to our church. My older daughter, Dana, welcomed Alysa and asked, "Do you want to sit with me?" After church we met the Conselyeas and made a dinner date. We loved them all from the beginning.

My younger daughter, Andrea, and Alysa attended Springfield Christian Academy at Dixie Baptist Church. Both cheerleaders, they spent a lot of time together. As often happens with teenage girls, they became friends but had an edge of competition between them. Andrea, an organized, neat planner contrasted with Alysa, the free, spontaneous, messy one. I can picture Alysa bouncing around, cheering, giggling and laughing. She had this incredible sense of humor and a quiet sweetness at the same time.

Spirit Week at the academy created great excitement. Each day had a different theme and the kids dressed accordingly. Can you imagine five consecutive days of Halloween? They'd find, borrow or beg clothes and props for "Western Day" or "Fifties Day." The girls participated wholeheartedly. Parents allied their enthusiasm with the kids' at the final pep rally the day before homecoming. Linda, getting into the spirit of things, came in one of Alysa's cheerleading outfits. She looked terrific and the young guys' chins dropped to their chests. Alysa was a little ticked that her mom got so much attention.

The Conselyeas went all out for Alysa's sixteenth birthday party. They catered a ton of Italian food and invited kids and their parents alike. Games, food and fun were in abundance. These kids from SCA didn't dance or go to movies so they made their own fun. One of their favorite, harmless pranks—draping lawns and trees with toilet paper—grew to monstrous proportions. To be "t.p.'d" meant status or notoriety. Teachers, parents—no one was spared. One of the school's counselors was a strict disciplinarian. To say he had zero rapport with the kids overstates his popularity. That night the kids decided that he would be their target.

Unfortunately, he heard and saw what was happening on his property and he bolted outside furiously, raving-mad. He started chasing kids and they went every which way. He finally grabbed Alysa and marched her to his car to report her, in person, to her parents. She opened the car door while the car was beginning to accelerate and rolled away collecting dirt and leaves in the process. She rendezvous'd with the other culprits and they sped to her home, arriving before the irate teacher.

Still at the party and privy to their planned antics, we parents reacted with surprise to Alysa and her friends when they burst through the door. The expressions on their faces said, "We're dead meat!" Wide-eyed and scared to death they hoped for some support from their parents.

When the teacher arrived, Dave invited him in and said, "Have some chicken!" He listened to the counselor's indignant tirade and with assurances that the kids would be reprimanded, he smoothed the old bird's feathers and doused his flaming anger. After all, they're just kids, and it's just toilet paper....

The girls would fool around at cheering practice. Although they had the gym to themselves, they still practiced wearing modest, baggy sweats. As a joke, someone's pants would be gripped from behind and yanked to her ankles. Now, I'm not saying Alysa did it, but if pranky things occurred, Alysa probably instigated it. Once a mother witnessed it and came unglued. I thought she should get a life. I think practical jokes, an inherited trait on the Rivers' side of the family, enhanced Alysa's liveliness. Dad Rivers, Linda, and Alysa are expert prank practitioners.

When Alysa became ill it was devastating. A vibrant, active, delightful young woman crushed to silence and immobility. To think that a simple virus caused it. It could have been one of my girls. My daughter Dana gave birth to her first baby the week Alysa got sick. The joy I knew with a new grandchild totally contrasted to the horror Linda experienced. I knew I had to be there for Linda—to encourage her. It turned out that she encouraged me.

Linda maintained a no-quit attitude and an enduring faith. My husband Tom and I would visit Alysa in the hospital, but we'd leave feeling quite helpless. There was nothing we could do or say, but we didn't want Linda and Dave to feel deserted.

For me the most devastating event occurred when the doctors recommended that Linda and Dave "pull the plug." They said there was no hope for Alysa and that she would never survive. Most people value the opinions of doctors and usually accept their knowledgeable advice. I wondered if everyone who knew Alysa was foolish to keep on hoping otherwise.

At that very hospital visit, we found Dave and Linda on their knees crying and praying. They were going to continue to trust in the Lord and depend on his power—not the doctors' opinions. Forget the specialists. They believed that until God says it's finished, it isn't finished. We left in distress. But we also came away in awe. Andy and Sylvia Rivers and Linda and Dave were not going to accept the wisdom of mere men.

I felt privileged to be one of their friends. They both devoted themselves to the care of Alysa. They did not eat, sleep or work. Alysa became the total focus of their lives. They had to have the empowering of the Holy Spirit. People could not withstand that ordeal in their own strength.

It made me evaluate what I do on a day to day basis—the trivialities that seem important. I take so much for granted. I do what I want to do and never think about the automatic. Swallowing and breathing are not tasks that I put on my "to do" list. The situation made me aware that I need to thank God daily for every nuance of my being. I wiggle my toes, open my eyes, bend my knees and lift my hands. They are all God's miracles.

I've learned to be more compassionate to people who are hurting or confined or limited. When I saw Alysa trapped in a body and mind that didn't work, my own problems became insignificant.

When I was thirteen my mother and I attended a Pentecostal revival. There were different speakers each night. One night a very strange-looking man took the platform. His clothes hung on

125

his body. His craggy, lined face was too large and his ears protruded oddly. I felt sorry for him. I wondered how he could get in front of people and not be embarrassed. After he spoke I learned non-judgmental compassion.

The minute his wonderful, expressive, kind voice sounded, he transformed right in front of my eyes. He spoke of the unconditional love of God. I decided at that moment that I wanted that kind of love in my life. I asked God to give me just a touch of what he gave that man. And he did.

CHAPTER TWELVE

Uncle Marc came in one last time to see Alysa—saddened that he never saw her awake during his six-day stay. Carrie Komisarz visited and presented Alysa with a stuffed animal that resembled a duck. But it also looked like a platypus. It was dubbed Plataduck and became the target of lighthearted jokes among the staff.

"If that yellow duck had any self respect, he'd volunteer to be duck a l'orange in the hospital cafeteria."

And, "That there animal is a throwback of nature. Its mama's flight path must have veered over Australia and she tarried too long in the weeds!"

The little animal was put to some good use. Often it would be an armrest for Alysa or as a divider to keep her many tubes from tangling. Sometimes when Alysa would have a washcloth on her forehead, the duck would be lying next to her with a washcloth on its forehead, too. The levity balanced the tragic seriousness of the situation to all involved.

The "Phantom of the Opera" tape was playing when Ken came to see his Sweetie. The nurses always chose to play Phantom instead of the mostly Christian artists' selections available.

He learned that Alysa was going back on Vancomycin because of bacteria found in her urine and her sputum—despite the protests of Alysa's parents. It appeared that the doctors waited until Dave and Linda were absent to approach Ken with their questions and concerns.

The resident somewhat apologetically told Ken, "I know the family doesn't want Alysa on Vancomycin, but it's what we have to use to fight the bacteria."

"I can assure you that Dave and Linda won't be pleased."

Next, an allergist spoke up, "The parents seem to think Alysa is allergic to Dilantin, too. What do you think?"

"We have it documented in our journals. She will develop redness, a rash and high fevers."

"Well, it probably wasn't dosed correctly. It just has to be started slowly," he said assuredly.

"I don't think so," Ken disagreed, shaking his head.

The Pentobarbital drip was stopped, again, on October 9. Alysa was trying to wake up. Her eyes fluttered and her nostrils flared.

That morning, she received hugs, love and excited conversation from her family. Then in the afternoon she had a coughing fit, had to be suctioned and bagged. Her blood oxygen had dropped to the mid-70's. Ken arrived just after the drama had ceased. Dr. Mattis, the infectious disease doctor, was in the room.

"We've stopped the Vancomycin. We think it probably caused the red man's rash."

"Imagine that," Ken said under his breath.

Dr. Baskin, the next doctor to have Ken's ear asked, "Do you think everyone is okay with using Dilantin?"

"Well, it's okay with me, but I'm not the one who makes the decisions. You have to ask Dave and Linda."

"Also, the pulmonologists recommend that she be trached again. How do the parents feel about that?"

"Look, I'm just Alysa's boyfriend. I can't answer these questions for you. Please talk to the Conselyeas."

When Linda and Dave showed up around 7:00 p.m., Ken was anxiety-ridden. "Hey, we've got to talk," he told them.

"Okay. Let's go to the waiting area, away from you-know-who's listening ears," Dave suggested. They never spoke negatively in front of Alysa.

Ken began. "I don't know why the doctors are asking me all this stuff. They seem to wait until you guys are gone."

"They do," Linda agreed. "I've even seen them duck into

stairwells when they see us coming. They avoid us at all cost," she said, fuming.

"So, what's up? What did they say tonight?" Dave directed the conversation back on track.

Ken related the comments and questions about Vancomycin, Dilantin and the trache. Then they went back to Alysa's bedside where Dave had planned to catch the vice presidential debates on Alysa's pullover TV. Laneen had chosen this time for one of her orchestrated visits. Her desire was to read scripture, then sing and have prayer in her orderly, engineering manner. Dave appreciated her kindheartedness. She did leave in time for him to catch the last half of the debates. He thought Jack Kemp was much better VP material than Al Gore.

The next morning during his pre-work visit, Ken was the lucky receiver of the doctors' tidings.

"We think Alysa has pneumonia and we are putting her back on the Vancomycin in spite of the rash. We'll give her Seldane to temper the effects."

Here we go again, Ken thought.

"Also, there appears to be seizure activity; therefore, we've put her on Dilantin. She'll have another EEG this afternoon."

Sirens went off in Ken's head. Linda is not going to be a happy camper. He absorbed the information and wrote it in the journal. He spent his remaining few moments holding Alysa's hand and caressing her cheek. "I love you. Get well, Pumpkinhead," he whispered.

Shortly after Ken left, Linda arrived and flipped open the journal. She read Ken's entry and she freaked. Alysa is on Dilantin!

"Call Dr. Baskin," she told Karen, the day nurse. I want to talk to her."

Karen returned and reported, "I reached Dr. Baskin and gave her your message. She couldn't talk to you now but said she'd be here in a few hours."

"Thanks, Karen."

Dr. Baskin was the only doctor at this hospital who was courteous or brave enough to talk to Linda and Dave—on occasion. The two had developed a respectful rapport. She stopped in as promised.

"Hello, Linda. I've decreased the Dilantin. You were right. It did spike fevers and cause an additional rash."

"I really do know about Alysa's reactions. We've been through all of this already," Linda reminded the doctor—when she really wanted to shout why didn't you listen to me?

"We've scheduled an EEG for later this afternoon and this could be our definitive EEG after stopping the drip."

"Linda, Ken's mom, and I will be spending time in the chapel praying for those results," Linda told her.

"Well, it couldn't hurt," the doctor said skeptically.

"But it most certainly can help. Second Chronicles 16:12 admonishes the king: 'Though his disease was severe, even in his illness he did not seek help from the Lord, but only from the physicians.' I want to seek the Lord's help."

Lamar, a gregarious, large, black Jehovah's Witness minister administered this EEG. Before he scooted the two Lindas from the room he said, "I'll be praying for her, too, Miss Linda."

"I know you will. Thanks, Lamar," Linda said, patting his large, capable hand.

At 5:30 p.m. the resident bore the good news. "Mrs. Conselyea, Alysa is out of status epilepticus."

"Praise the Lord!" Linda and Linda Two said simultaneously, while clasping hands and dancing around in circles.

Dr. Baskin called the nurses' station and wanted Linda brought to the phone.

"Linda. I'm just thrilled over the EEG report," she began. "We will discontinue the Pentobarbitol drip. And we'll remove the respiratory tube."

"This is all an answer to prayer," Linda claimed.

"I'll be watching Alysa closely these next few days," she said. "We'll talk tomorrow. G'bye."

It was surprising when a surgeon stepped in the next morning to check Alysa's trache site. It was puffy and discolored.

"Why are you looking at the trache site, Doctor?" Linda asked.

"A tracheostomy has been ordered and I wanted to see if the infection would interfere with the procedure."

Linda, somewhat bewildered responded, "We haven't discussed this with Dr. Baskin. She wants Alysa off the respirator. We haven't given our okay, either. So, I don't know what you are talking about!"

Tactics were delayed, and a week later the re-traching of Alysa resurfaced. Dr. Forentino from pulmonology had cornered Ken that morning.

"I heard that the family has agreed to the trache. But, they haven't signed the consent forms. Would you please have them page me when they come in today?"

When Ken got to work, he called Linda and told her what the doctor had said.

"I don't know where they get their information," she said to Ken.

"They sure like to talk to me."

"I wish they'd talk to us about what they're doing. We are always the last to find out."

"You're to page Dr. Forentino when you go in."

"I will. How did Alysa look this morning?"

"She was awake and shook her head yes and no. She looked good. She had a bath and her hair looked pretty. Good vitals. No fever, too."

"Good. I'll be there around 8:30. See you at 5:00?"

"Sure will. See you then."

"Bye now."

Linda paged Dr. Forentino upon her arrival. He came to see her.

"I'm not sure where you get your information, but my husband and I have not yet consented to a trache," she began.

"Well, let me tell you what we think. From her breathing treatments we can tell that she doesn't have full-lung capacity. The induced coma knocked the strength out of her. She still isn't able to cough. All of these signs tell us that she needs to remain on the respirator and it isn't wise to continue with the oral respiratory tube. I would like for you to consider these things; discuss it with your husband and get back to me."

Linda called Dave at work and they weighed the pros and cons. Always wanting the best for their daughter, they decided to pray about it and make their decision that evening.

At 8:00 Dave and Linda both signed the consent form for the second tracheostomy their daughter would endure. It felt like another step backwards, but they trusted God for his ways. They turned to their daughter.

"Lys, Honey. The doctors think it's best that you be put back on the ventilator full time with another tracheostomy. We want you to be breathing comfortably, so we said okay," Dave said.

"It will just be until your lungs get strong again," Linda said encouragingly.

Changing the subject, he handed her a form and a pen and said, "Lysa, this is a form for you to get an absentee ballot. Let me help you and we'll sign your name. Wouldn't want you to not be able to vote, would we?"

"Lysa, I'm going to read 1 Samuel, chapter one. And then your Dad's going to pray."

Afterwards, they told Alysa good night. "I'm going to put your Sandi Patti tape in for you, Sweetie," Dave said knowing Sam, the night nurse, would have it whipped out and "Phantom" playing before he get down the hallway.

Thursday, October 24
Day 165

7:00 a.m. Both Lindas here. Nurse Samantha thought Alysa had partial seizure this morning. They didn't give her anything. Lasted one to two minutes. Anesthesiologist in. Alysa supposed to go down for trache surgery at 9:30, then 10:00, 10:30, 11:00 and finally at 11:20 she went for surgery. 12:05 Surgery finished. Doctor said trache site infected and worse on the inside. Sent a culture to the lab. 12:20 Ken writing. Went to get sandwich while Alysa getting fixed up in her room. 12:40 Alysa's eyes open. Looks great. We had a great prayer time. I love her so much! 2:00 H.R.= 89, B.O.=90, Resp=24. I'm leaving at 2:10.

7:30 DJC/LRC here. Alysa looks good. H.R. 110, B.O. 98, Resp. 15. Temp. 99. She feels warm. Eyes staring but reacting to light. 7:45 Leann and Deborah in to help reposition Alysa. They tell me her skin still looks real good. All the nurses were fighting to take care of Alysa today. Leann won. Tomorrow may be the day that she gets moved. 8:15 Respiratory tech in to suction through the trache. Sam in to say hi. 9:20 Sam and Linda had a long talk. 9:50 Mom has been reading to Alysa—one of those girls' books. I took MY blood pressure and it was 115/69! 10:30 Mom gave Alysa a super shave job and full body wash. 11:00 Sam taking over for Leann. Both of them started working on Alysa's trache. New gauze and neck strap. She looks beautiful! I gave her a leg and foot massage. 11:45. Resp. in for suctioning. We're putting everything in bags getting ready for tomorrow's move. 12:30 a.m. After Bible readings and prayers, Linda and I are going home. H.R.=90, B.O.=98. Sleeping now.

On Day 166, Alysa started her residence in room 335, #1, East. It was the first time she was not in a private room. Her roommate, Virginia, was blind and was suffering from a leg amputation. The poor lady screamed in pain, which upset Alysa terribly. Linda noticed that Alysa's fingers on both hands were moving rhythmically and her eyes were darting. By 4:00 her eyes settled down, but her lower jaw jerked up and down.

"Do you think she needs some medication?" Linda asked the nurse.

"I'll check the chart and see what Dr. Baskin has ordered."

Later, Stephanie Baskin called in and talked to Linda. "I really don't think it is seizure activity. I'll keep checking on her," she said.

The following day Alysa was sweating and twitching both arms simultaneously. She still had some mouth movement. Grandma Rivers observed her behavior.

"This reminds me of the beginning. Is it ever going to stop?"

"Remember, Mom, these are like muscle spasms. It doesn't necessarily mean she is having seizures."

"I know, I know. My poor baby. She has suffered through so much. I guess I thought that after the induced coma, she'd come out fine—like before any of this happened. It's just a disappointment. I know God won't let us down. Linda, if you'll fill this basin with water for me, I'm going to cool her down. The sweat is just dripping down her neck."

Linda rummaged through the nightstand. "Okay. Where have they hidden all the washcloths?" Supplies found, task begun. Another day caring and loving Alysa.

Dr. Abraham called on his car phone on the way home from the airport to check on his former patient.

"Alysa, Honey," Linda said. "It's Dr. Abraham calling to say hi."

Surprisingly alert, Alysa eyes shone with excitement and she lifted her arms for an over-the-wire embrace.

Interview with Linda Beaudoin

The aroma of spicy, bubbling, tomato sauce invaded the rooms of Linda Beaudoin's tri-level house on the northeast side of Detroit. All the kids—Ken, Matt and his wife Nikki, Carrie and Kelly—were expected to show up for spaghetti night. As a single parent for the past 11 years, Linda was accustomed to nurturing, caring and providing for her close-knit offspring. After her divorce, she reinstated her maiden name, Beaudoin.

Linda recalls those times:

When Kelly was in elementary school, the counselor insisted I come for a meeting. She knew all four of my kids, and I had met her on other occasions. I walked in for the conference, and she said she wanted to shake my hand. She was amazed that my children came from a broken home and insisted that she could always tell which kids were in single-parent homes. She congratulated me for a job well done. Without a husband and father in the home, I guess I just gave more attention to my children. Really, I was just blessed with good kids.

Ken, my oldest, at age 23 moved into a house down the block, but when Alysa got sick, we sold that house and he moved back home. Kelly was a senior in high school and was the valedictorian. Carrie was living at home, too, when Ken and Alysa first started dating. Alysa was like one of the family. She camped here about 90% of the time. She would sleep over, on the couch, and she and I would solve the world problems over coffee in the mornings. Half of Ken's clothes ended up at her grandmother's house because she'd borrow them and wear them home.

Alysa had a goodness about her. Always happy, she just beamed with energy and enthusiasm. We noticed something was different about her before she got really sick. The day before Mother's Day she was over at Nikki's, my daughter-in-law's, and she was irritable. She was very short with Nikki, and she was talking a mile a minute.

We were not surprised the next day when Ken called and said that Alysa was in the emergency room. We all went over to support him: not because it was his girlfriend, but because it was Alysa. I couldn't just stand by and see a 21-year-old girl in need, and I wanted to help out all I could.

After that first week, I pretty much became the night shift person. I wanted to help relieve the burden that Linda and Dave had in their 24-hour vigil. I would go to the hospital around 10:00 p.m. so they could go to Sylvia's to sleep. If someone wasn't with Alysa, the hospital would have put her in restraints, and Linda and Dave abhorred that idea. During her coma she didn't just lie in bed. She did 360's constantly. Her arms, legs and whole body would thrash. We were both bruised from the bouts of trying to keep her in the bed. IV-wired, trached and catheterized, she would become entangled in a web of medical tubes and wires. She would fight for hours upon hours. One night the urinary catheter, or Foley, had to be replaced five times.

When the respiratory therapists would come in to administer her treatments, I would leave for five minutes to have my own "respiratory treatment." My smoking is something I've tried to eliminate, but without success. On one of those occasions, I returned to the room to discover that after changing the sheets and getting Alysa settled, they had restrained her. It was heartbreaking to see Alysa tug continuously at those restraints. Angered, I called Dave to tell him what happened. He returned to the hospital and had the restraints removed.

The restraints were not for meanness; their work was made easier by restraining patients when they were understaffed, which appeared to be most of the time. For that reason, Linda, and all of us, became pretty proficient with what we called our spa treatments. It was important to all of us that Alysa be kept looking nice. We washed her hair, applied lotion to her body, washed her and shaved her legs and underarms. We had to clean her and the bedding after bowel movements, too. Her dignity was uppermost in our minds. These things would not have been done expediently by the staff, if at all.

We would talk to her as if she were talking back. We did not talk over or about her. We were told that people in comas do hear, so we would just tell her what's been going on in our daily lives. Alysa was supposed to do Kelly's hair for her prom. Instead, on prom night, Kelly and her date went to the hospital to see Alysa and tell her their plans for the evening.

Even though she didn't respond, I'm sure that Alysa heard her mother's voice. She was calmed by known voices. Her mother's voice especially soothed her. We would read to her and play music. One morning Amy Grant's "A Joyful Heart Is Good Medicine" was playing. Alysa started sobbing and I sobbed along with her.

Linda and Dave were always so concerned about me. They knew I had health complications from having experienced septic shock. Also, my rheumatoid arthritis acts up. They constantly asked me how I felt, and considered my pain and comfort. They showed that kind of concern with everyone in the hospital. Dave would bring in food for people, and Linda would bring birthday cakes and treats for the staff. They would thank me for being there every time. They would thank the staff for doing their jobs. And they demonstrated such compassion with Ken.

Linda and Dave realized the strong commitment that Ken had made to Alysa. They honored that by including him in their discussions of Alysa's care. Ken was seeing Alysa before work, on his lunch hour and again after work. Dave once gave Ken an out if he wanted it. "Ken, don't you think you should consider getting on with your life?" he had asked him. Ken said that his life entwined with Alysa's because he loved her.

When Alysa was diagnosed "status epilepticus," Ken became despondent and depressed. He worked, paid all of my household bills and spent all his spare time at Alysa's bedside. He had to see a doctor himself because he was so distraught. When Kelly saw Ken crying, she told Carrie, who in turn became emotional. Carrie was so upset observing her brother's depression that she moved out of the house.

I had twelve years of Catholic education, knew all the devotions and masses in Latin and English, but I didn't know how to pray. Linda and Dave taught me how to pray to our Lord. We would gather around Alysa's bed, hold hands and talk to God. They always thanked and praised God. They didn't just beseech him for help in their great time of need. They also gave me my prized possession: a woman's devotional Bible.

That night when I heard my tenderhearted son crying in his room, sobbing, I got down on my knees and gave my son back to God for his good keeping. I realized that I couldn't help his hurt. With Kelly bawling and Carrie in hysterics at work, I got down on my knees again and said, "Okay, Lord, I guess you want them all!" A passage in my Bible confirmed my action. Anxious to share it, I got dressed, called Sylvia and went to the hospital. We wrote it in the journal.

The journals are another amazing part of the documentation of Alysa's illness. They began as record keeping for medicines and medical evaluations. As one of us would come in, we could read what had happened before our shift. As the days and months progressed, the entries became more of a personal diary written to Alysa. When Alysa is fully recovered, Lord willing, she won't have the regret of having missed a year and a half of her life. It's all there: a recorded gift of love.

At first I was real bent on Why? A beautiful young girl, strong Christian parents…why did this happen to them? In time, I realized that God knows what he is doing. He has a reason. He had Alysa on a mission and sometimes I feel guilty that my coming to know him is a result of that mission. Overall I learned that prayer is the answer.

And Ken has taught me so much. I thought I was proud of his good grades, his sports honors and academic accolades, but nothing has made me so proud compared to the man I see now. The doctors say that husbands walk away from wives with illnesses less devastating than Alysa's. This is definitely a love story.

Interview with Ken Komisarz

Soft-spoken, articulate, serious, and solid—these words describe Ken Komisarz, Alysa's boyfriend. He's a good-looking twenty-seven-year-old man who knows exactly who he is. After acquiring a materials and logistics degree from Michigan State University, he worked as a buyer for Copper and Brass. His current job is with ITT Automotive as a Supplier Development Engineer. In that position, he travels around the country to oversee suppliers' production and to conduct on-site quality audits. He was working the former job during Alysa's illness, when he made his daily trips to see her.

Ken shares his memories:

I am the oldest of four children. I have one brother and two sisters. It was my sister-in-law who played matchmaker and fixed me up with Alysa. She told me there was this really neat girl at beauty school who was pretty, fun and available. To Alysa she presented me as the strong, silent type but an "okay" guy. With

137

such glowing attributes, how could we refuse to be introduced?

We met on my birthday, October 31, 1994, but didn't have a date until a couple of weeks later. We went to the Big Fish Two for dinner and to see the movie "Interview With A Vampire" afterwards. What a romantic first date.

That first date movie choice must not have been a detriment, because our relationship flourished. I was attracted to Alysa's outgoing manner. She was bubbly, and she made people around her feel happy. She was generous, thoughtful and very attractive.

We got to know each other's family and friends and included each other in our own interests and pursuits. I had never thought much about religion and God, but if you're with Alysa, the subject comes up all the time. She is a woman of faith and she was always concerned about where I stood with the Lord. We had conversations and debates to the point that she had piqued my interest.

I was raised Catholic, but I was never confirmed. I was not a big church-goer. Alysa would take me to her church—and that was a real trip! I thought church was ceremony and ritual. Not at her church. Pastor Jim would preach in his meaningful and heartfelt style and I was captivated. We even met Pastor Jim for lunch one day and he explained how his church doctrine differs from that of the Catholic Church.

When Alysa started to get sick, her desire for my being saved became passionate. I can remember sitting on the swings in the park on the day that she first went to the emergency room. She was spiritually hyper, if there is such a thing. I knew I wasn't going to be forced into being saved. It had to be a logical decision for me.

The third night that Alysa was in Bellville, Dave and Linda had gone and I was alone with her. I had told myself that when I accepted the Lord, it wasn't going to be at a moment of weakness, or for selfish reasons. I didn't want to be needing him. I thought I should accept Christ when nothing was wrong in my life. But it didn't happen that way.

I was next to Alysa's bed and I bowed my head and said silently, "Oh, Lord Jesus, I want you in my heart and my life. Please forgive my sins. And please heal Alysa. Amen." There was nothing I wouldn't do for Alysa, but I was doing this for myself. Now, this is going to sound weird, but I had a feeling that someone was standing directly behind me. It scared me, it was so strong. I even turned around to look, but no one was there. That prayer of acceptance was my covenant with God alone.

People have questioned my sticking around all this time. It is completely foreign to me that anyone would leave. If you love the person, there's nothing else you can do. I couldn't live with myself if I split. I can't fathom how someone could leave. I was reading a woman's magazine—there wasn't anything else around to read—and there was an interview with the wife of Christopher Reeves. She was called a saint. She disagreed and said that a saint chooses a lifestyle. She said that she had no choice and would never have chosen this life for her husband. She just reacts.

That's what you do. You just do what you have to do. I have to believe that other people would do the same. Even with all the good that has come from this situation, I can't be generous enough to say that it was worthwhile. I hated Alysa's apparent suffering and would rather that it never happened. If I could take it back, I would.

Alysa was so fortunate to have the love and support of her parents. They were steadfast in their faith and based their decisions on that faith. It was a lesson to me on how to handle a difficult situation with an ill child. I only hope I could handle it as well, if I ever have to.

Interview with Carrie and Kelly Komisarz

Ken's sisters, Carrie and Kelly Komisarz are alike and different at the same time. Five years separate them in age, but a strong sense of family joins them. Both are attractive, with dark hair and eyes. Kelly's intensity and seriousness contrast with Carrie's more casual joie de vivre.

Diminutive seems too big a word to describe the tiny Kelly, but it fits. Carrie's flair for fashion and hip hair style denotes her more casual lifestyle view. One thing they definitely have in common is their love for Alysa.

It didn't start out that way:

"I met her for the first time on a trip up north with Matt and Nikki," said Carrie. "Nikki had invited Alysa and me to go along. Nikki and Alysa were in the back seat, kidding and cutting up the entire three hours. I had a headache and, actually, they were loud and annoying."

"But you changed your mind," Kelly said in Alysa's defense.

"Yeah, I did. I got to know her that weekend and we had a lot of fun. After that, she started coming over and hanging out a lot. I grew to love her."

"You influenced my opinion of her," Kelly stated. "I expected not to like her, but when I met her at Christmastime, she was great. She didn't treat me like a kid. I was only 15 then. She'd sit and talk to me on my level about school and life. We bonded quickly."

Carrie added, "That's right. She became like a sister. Since she was an only child, she loved being with all of us. She adopted us and we adopted her. She was always cooking and making us special coffee. Even though she was a church-goer, she was so happy, peppy and even silly."

"She'd stay overnight and blow-dry my hair before I'd go to school. That was pretty neat—to have my own hair stylist," said Kelly.

"Alysa is 15 days younger than I, so we called each other 'big sister' and 'little sister.' I told her that she should respect her elders. Me!" Carrie said. "Everything seemed so perfect."

"Then she got sick. I knew something was wrong," Kelly agreed. "My friend, Melissa, went to Bardha Salon for Alysa to do her hair. She was embarrassed afterwards that she didn't have enough money to pay Alysa the full amount. Normally, Alysa wouldn't have minded at all. That night when Ken and Alysa were here watching TV, Alysa told me in a snippy voice that Melissa didn't pay her. I was shocked! A little later Alysa came to my room and apologized. She said she wasn't feeling well. That happened right before her first seizure."

"That day sure sticks out in my memory," Carrie said. "I work at Bellville as a Physical Therapy Patient Transporter, and I was working there when Ken brought Alysa into the ER. I went in to see her. She kept saying, 'I had a seizure? I can't believe I had a seizure.'"

Kelly chimed in, "We all came to the hospital. It was so scary. We were all bawling. We wondered if something happened at the Redken convention to cause the seizure. I was too upset to go to school the next day. I can remember Alysa repeated over and over 'just a little piece of life.' It didn't make any sense to me."

"While she was at Bellville I'd check on her throughout the day. Once she screamed my name when she saw me. Another time I heard her moaning. By then she was heavily sedated. It was horrible. I didn't want to go into her room. I'd sit and talk with my brother in the waiting room. I just wanted to be there for him."

"I didn't go to Bellville much. I was there that first night, but I didn't go in to see her," Kelly admitted. "I do remember going to Oakhill Memorial. It was prom night. Alysa was supposed to have fixed my hair. That was two weeks after her first seizure. I had thought she'd be well in time for my hair appointment. Instead, she was totally out of it. I held her hand and thought maybe she knew who I was. It made me feel better to be there."

"But it got harder for you," Carrie said.

"I know it's selfish," Kelly admitted, "but later on when she wasn't getting any better, I found it hard to go visit her."

"Tom and I would go," Carrie said, "and we'd find her trached, tied down and in a coma-like trance. I would get pretty emotional. I'd hold her hand, play the radio, read to her and help her mom wash her hair and shave her legs. We'd give her a "spa" treatment. I had to do something for her. I'd want to reach her. I'd reminisce aloud about funny things we'd done together, like when she was driving Ken's brand new Saturn. We were stopping at a light in the right turn lane. The car was a stick shift. She pushed the clutch by itself, and of course nothing happened. She let it up and slammed on the brake. The car pitched forward and the engine choked and died—deader than a doornail. The expression on her face was priceless. We both cracked up."

Kelly chided herself. "I had to force myself to go see her. I didn't want to hear anything bad. I didn't want to face a setback. I couldn't be strong like her parents. They were so positive. Linda would talk to Alysa like she was right there. They are the most caring people I've ever met. Linda and Dave were so sensitive to other people. He'd make me feel better by changing the subject and talking about other things. He knew I cared about Alysa, and I think he knew I had trouble facing her situation."

Carrie agreed. "I know how Kelly felt. It helped me to do something for her or buy her a present. Something bright and cheery. Her rooms were so blah, they needed to be brightened up. I took her a goofy looking duck once, clothes, cards, and dried flowers. Kristin, a friend of mine at work, wanted to do something for her, too. She made a small Christmas tree for Alysa."

"I think her sickness made us all stronger and increased our faith," Kelly volunteered.

"She was so sick that the doctors wanted to turn the machines off. It seemed hopeless. I never prayed so much in my life." Carrie concluded.

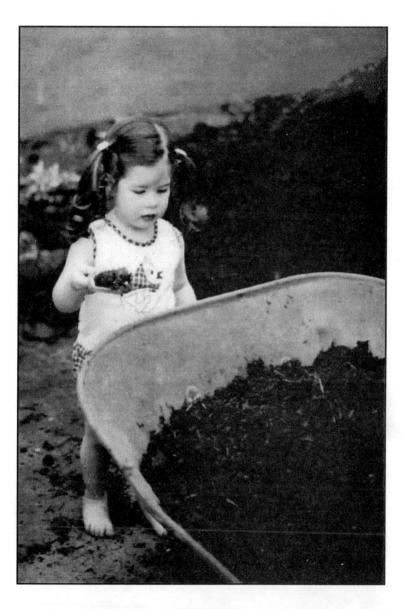

**Spreading manure on Grandma's garden doesn't
faze two-an-a-half-year-old Alysa.**

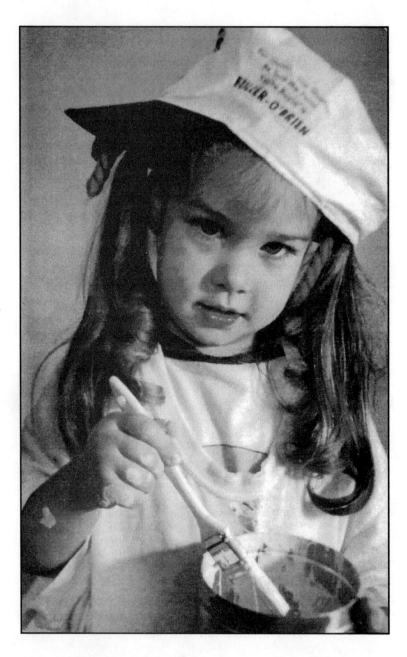

Four-year-old paint mate, Alysa, proudly paints a wall to help Grandpa Rivers.

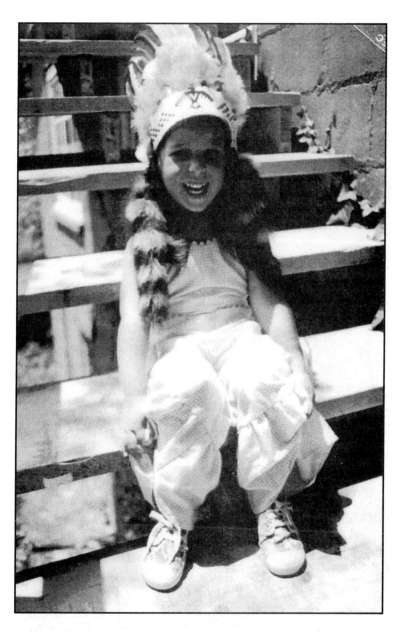

**Alysa wears her beloved Indian headdress
from Cherokee, North Carolina.**

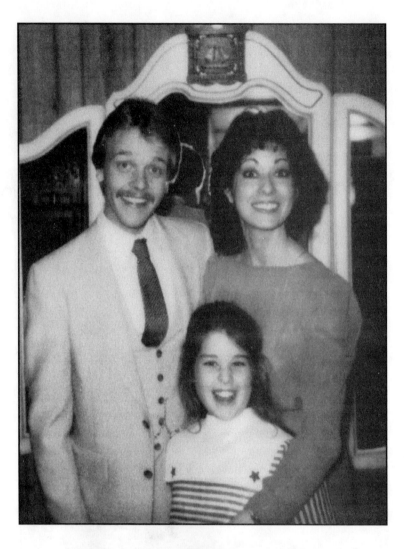

**Linda says "yes" to Dave's marriage proposal
in November 1983. The nine-year-old
Alysa granted her okay.**

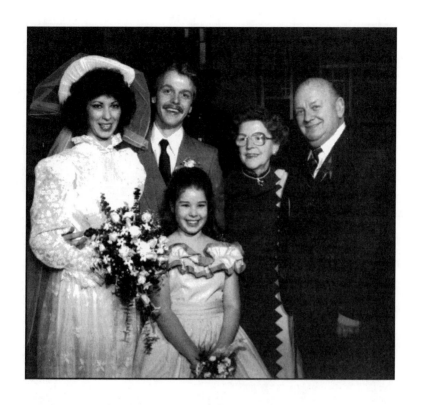

One month later Alysa serves as a flower girl
in her parent's wedding on Christmas Day.
The elder Conselyeas celebrate
the joining of the new family.

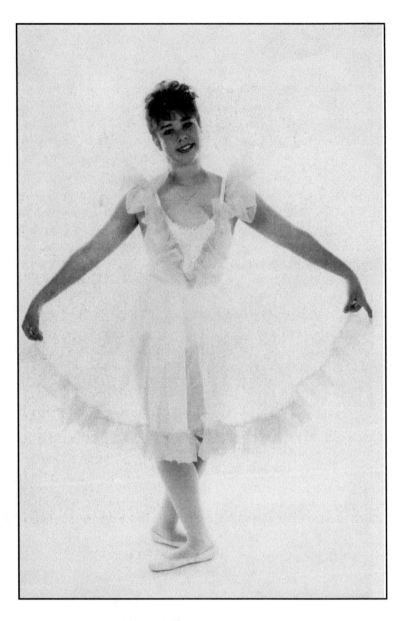

**Alysa, age 9, loved her dancing lessons
at Juliana's Academy of Dance.**

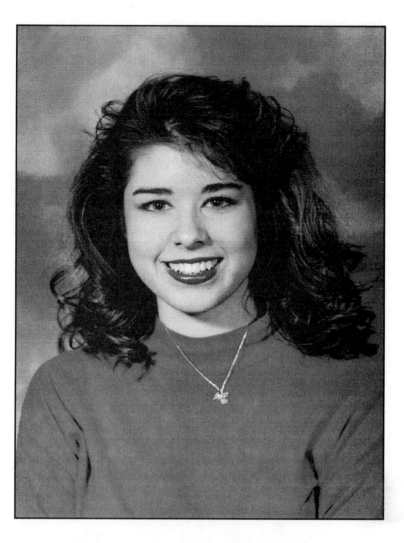

**Alysa wears her Sweet Sixteen pendant
as a junior in high school.**

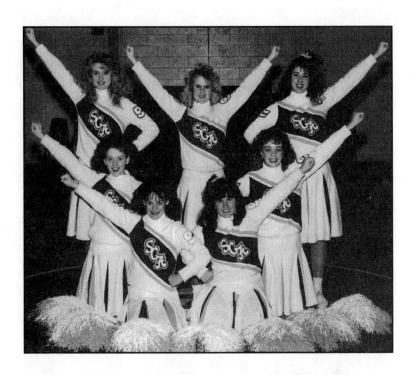

**Posing with the 1990-91 varsity cheerleading
squad at Springfield Christian School is
Alysa in the back row, far right.**

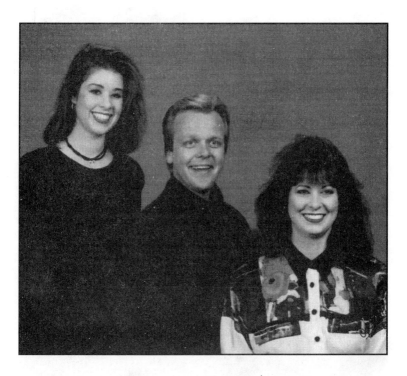

**Alysa, age 20, joins her parents, Linda and
Dave Conselyea, for a family portrait.**

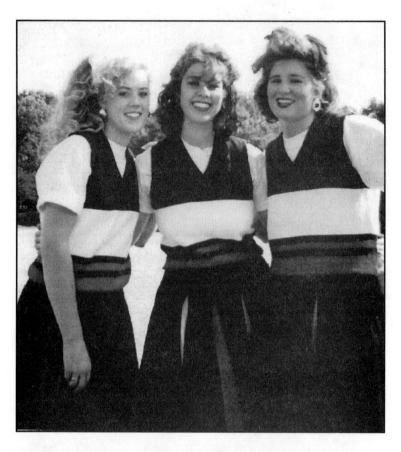

Cheerleading pals at Bob Jones University. Brandy Gilbert, Alysa and Stephanie Forester smile for the camera.

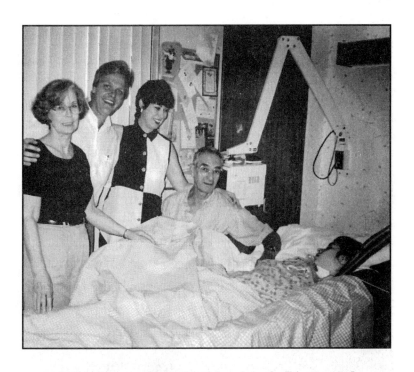

Sylvia Rivers, Dave, Linda and Andy Rivers tend to Alysa after her ICU scare at Oakhill Memorial.

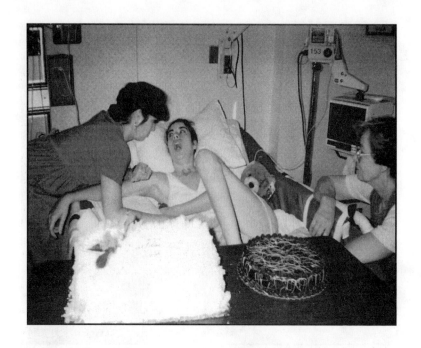

On August 29, 1996, the family pretended that all was well for Alysa's twenty-second birthday the following day.

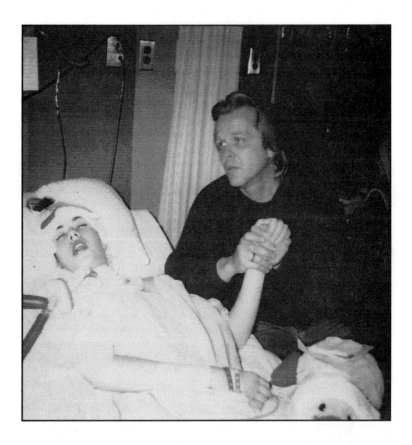

Dad Dave keeps his watchful vigil during one of Alysa's high fever bouts at St. Vincent's Hospital. The stuffed animal, Plataduck, sports a washcloth, too.

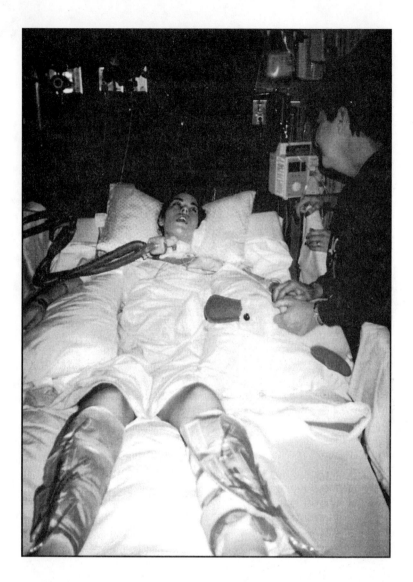

While at St. Vincent's, Alysa is kept up to date on family events by the caring Linda Beaudoin. Alysa wears her leg wraps and her "geisha" shoes and has a catatonic stare.

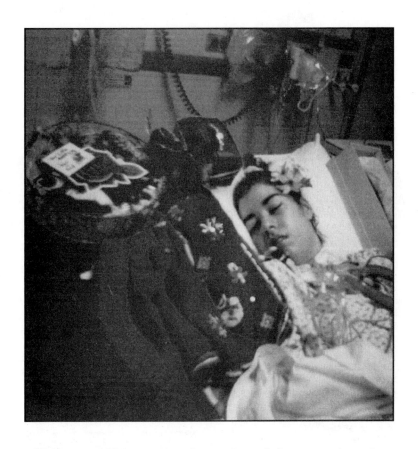

Christmas 1996, pneumonia sets in and the non-responsive Alysa spends a lonely day in ICU at Mid Town Hospital.

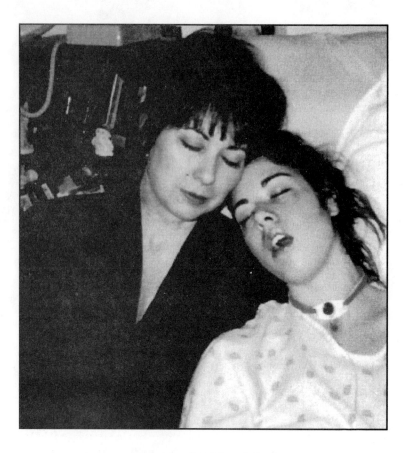

**A rare moment—double winks for mom
and daughter at Crooked Creek.**

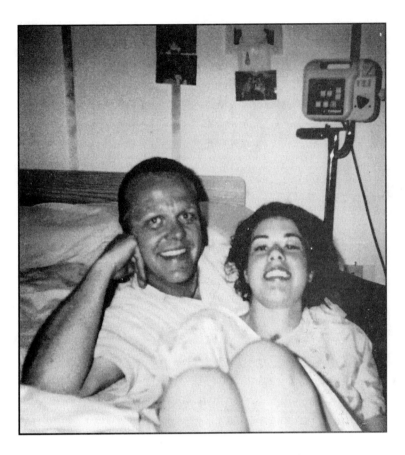

Pony-tailed dad with a responsive daughter—PTL!

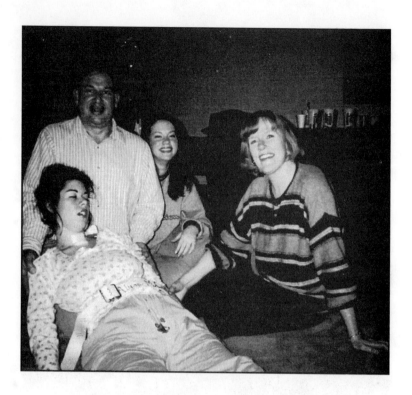

**Pete, Becky and Pat Toth relax after a strenuous
stand and sit exercise session with Alysa.**

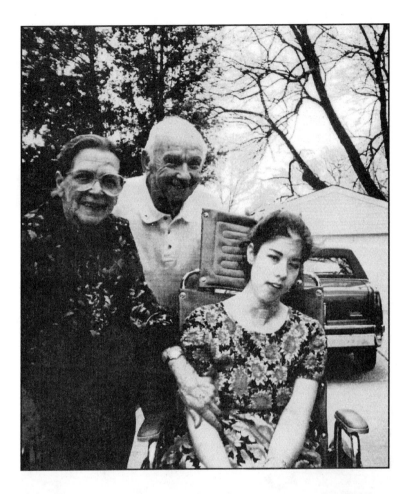

Mother's Day 1997, one year after the onset of her illness, Alysa takes her first trip out of Crooked Creek and makes a surprise visit to Grandma and Grandpa Conselyea's house. (Ralph Conselyea died August 31, 1999.)

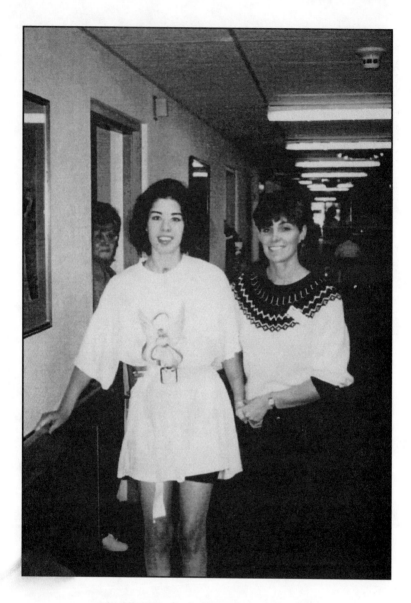

**Alysa's physical therapist assists her
in relearning how to walk.**

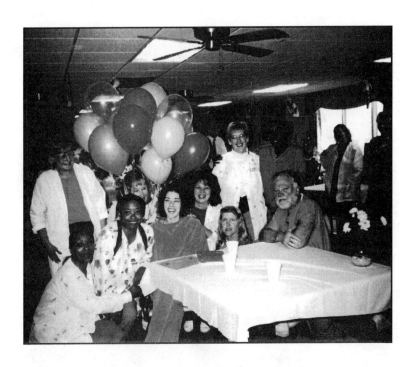

**Day 486, September 10, 1997,
is discharge day from Crooked Creek.**

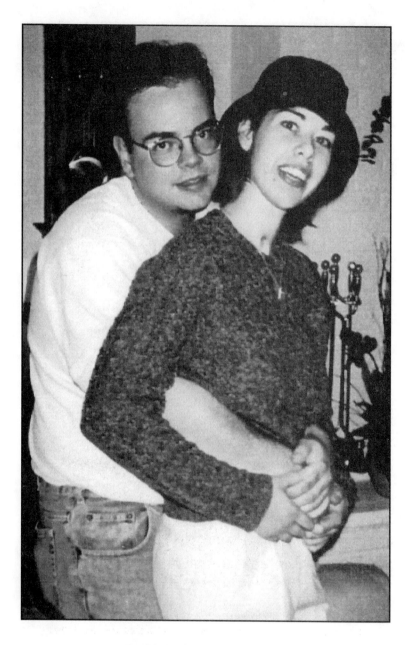

Happiness is coming home!

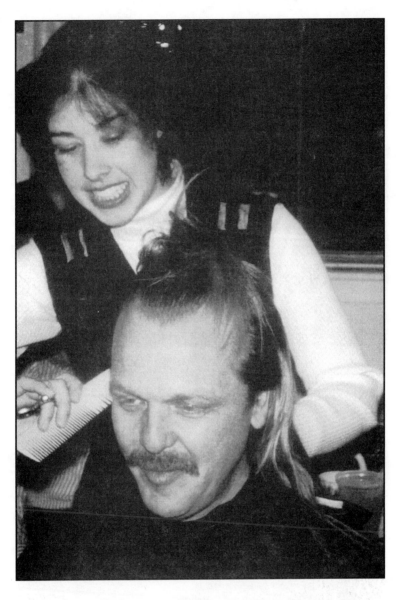

With an unsteady hand and with friends and family
watching, Alysa performs her first haircut—on Dad!
The audience cheers the loss of the ponytail.

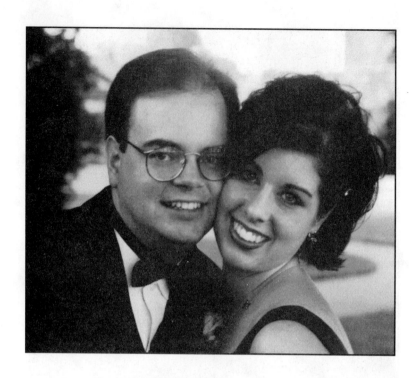

**Ken and Alysa become engaged at her
birthday party on August 29, 1999.**

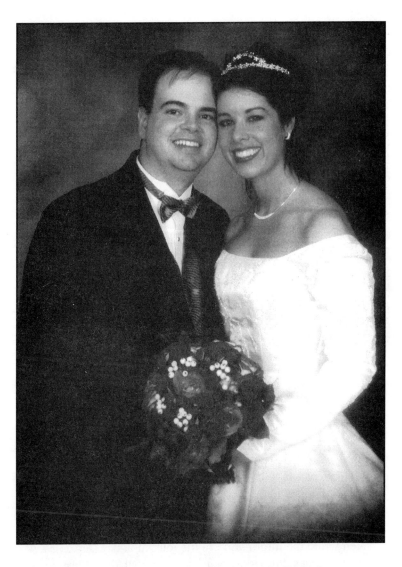

On December 30, 2000, Alysa Marie Conselyea
and Kenneth Komisarz were wed amid the tears and joy
of friends and loved ones who witnessed a miracle.

CHAPTER THIRTEEN

Ken stopped in before work on October 31, his 26th birthday. Alysa did not answer or acknowledge his unusual greeting.

"Good morning, Goldilocks! Someone curled your hair. Boy, you'd poop a purple Twinkie if you could see what it looks like. But that's okay," he said, twirling one of the curls between his fingers. "You'd look beautiful no matter what. It's really cold out today. Thirty-two degrees and a wind chill of zero. Old Man Winter is at the door!"

"Hello, Ken," the physician's assistant recognized Alysa's visitor. "Alysa is pretty sedated, as you can tell. It looks like she'll be on the vent a few more days. We're thinking of having her off for twelve hours and then back on for twelve hours. We'll see."

"Is there any more news on a low-level rehab for her?"

"We're still checking on that. Maybe Lakeland will take her."

Ken wrote the information in the journal under Day 172.

Alysa's eyes fluttered open and shut that day. She seemed awake when Ken read his birthday cards to her later that evening. This day had been one more holiday and birthday that Alysa unwillingly ignored. It also marked the two-year anniversary of when they first met.

Ken tried not to think too far into the future. But would Alysa be well this time next year? Would she even be alive? He was contemplating marriage. Trust in God, he told himself.

Saturday, November 2
Day 174

8:15 a.m. Good Morning, Sweetie! Ken's here for the day. Go Green! And Go White! Michigan, Go Blow! Spartans are going to do it today! Alysa looks good. Wide awake. B.O.=96, H.R.=121, Resp=13. 8:45 Blood ox. dropped to 88. They suctioned a lot of stuff out and she was fine. Lila came in to change her tube and put her on CPAP. Dr. Graves and P.A. Jerry Stephens came in and looked at her. He said no change, just trying to wean her off the vent. Started moving around 1:15, mostly mouth and eyes. Slight hand twitching. One more hour till Ativan. After one quarter of play, Michigan leads Michigan State 7 to 3. We were robbed of a touchdown reception, though. Mom was here for about an hour, but her hip started hurting and she went home to take a pain pill. 1:30 Temp=101.3. Put ice bag on her and gave Tylenol with her Phenobarb. Nurse wants to take blood, sputum and urine samples due to temp. Calling doctor about giving her Ativan while on CPAP. Mr. Presley came by and stayed 45 minutes. Small BM. Twitching off and on for about an hour. 2:00 Very still. May be sleeping. Michigan State 10, Michigan 28. Come on, Spartans! Off CPAP at 2:15. Alysa almost looked angry about going on SIMV (full vent). I guess she likes taking the breaths on her own and doesn't want the machine to do it for her. Good girl! She pursed her lips, turned her head and moved her left arm to the side of the bed. Lila gave Ativan, shot in the arm, at 2:30. Kelly just called and said she got her acceptance letter to MSU. Maybe she can help the football team! Temp=100.5 at 2:50. 3:50 Pulled her head away when I wiped her face. Also, moved arms to her belly. Sweaty now, feels hot. 4:15 Dr. Berto stopped by. Said they were waiting for Lakeland review. Marilyn is nurse until 7:00 a.m.

Mr. David Presley, the founder of the cosmetology school, made a surprising visit to see Alysa. Alysa had developed a fond relationship with the octogenarian when she attended his beauty school.

"You know, Alysa really has what it takes," he told Ken. "She has a great attitude toward her customers. She's one student who can make it in the beauty field. I sure hope she can get well and get back to it."

"Thank you for your compliments, sir. I really hope she can, too. It was so nice of you to come and visit her today. I know her parents will be disappointed that they missed you."

"You tell them they have a fine daughter. It's just a shame to see her like this," he said, shaking his head as he left the room.

November 5th was voting day. Jerry Stephens told Linda the new discovery. "We've got Alysa on a Heparin drip today. Alysa has developed a blood clot below her knee. Don't give her any massages or rub her body because we don't want it to break away."

"That's pretty dangerous, isn't it?"

"It could be, but the blood thinner should lessen any risk."

Linda knelt by the bed and prayed for the blood clot to dissolve.

Complications continued. Dr. Berto, one who never pulled any punches, informed Linda that Alysa could easily have died from status epilepticus. He was on call when he hurriedly, almost offhandedly, made that remark.

"Doctor, I'm not sure I'm glad that you shared that with me, but what's worse, look at Alysa."

Tears had welled up in Alysa's eyes and were leaking down her cheeks.

"We have never spoken negatively in Alysa's presence for that very reason," Linda said, pointing to her daughter.

The doctor looked but said nothing.

A catastrophe of another sort materialized late that night, according to Dave: four more years of Slick Willie.

The social worker who had been assigned to Alysa's case drew Linda aside to tell her of an upcoming meeting with the doctors about possible rehab.

"Someone from Grand Blanc will be coming to assess Alysa. Also, I know you have been wanting to talk to the doctors about some of your concerns. How about Tuesday?"

"Shirley, remember when we had that long talk and you said I should be doing something for myself? Not just live at the hospital day in and day out?"

Shirley nodded her head.

"Tuesday is my one day, in fact, my only morning that I do something special. That is my Bible Study Fellowship meeting and I try never to miss it. Can't the doctors meet on any other day but Tuesday?"

"I'll see what I can arrange," she promised.

"It's amazing that we can never corral the doctors, but when they deem it so, their time is more important than mine. Good luck!"

Dr. Baskin came in on Saturday, November 9. She had ordered that Alysa be weaned off the respirator. Ken was the one to receive her furor.

"Who discontinued the Ativan?" she asked Ken.

Before he could reply and while she was studying the chart, she blurted, "And Klonopin? Who wrote that order? What's going on here?"

She flipped the pages of the chart and saw that the pulmonologist had changed her orders—again. She spoke to Linda and Dave that night and shared her dissatisfaction with the other doctors. The Conselyeas, caught in the middle of the medical game playing and one-upsmanship, remained silent.

"I think that her weaning from the respirator should be much more aggressive and I shall advise that. I am the primary doctor in charge of Alysa. Besides, I think you should know that when we have our meeting on Thursday they intend to discuss discontinuing life support. Alysa is not brain dead. I'm totally against it," she concluded.

"Discontinuing life support?" Dave repeated.

"What did you say?" asked Linda.

"Oh, I guess I let their cat out of the bag. They are ready to give up on her. That's what this meeting is truly about—whether we keep Alysa dependent on life support."

"No way. Absolutely not. They are not going to discontinue life support for my daughter," Linda said with forceful conviction. Linda immediately turned to the phone—her link with her prayer support.

"Cindy? Linda. I'm fine. The doctors are considering pulling the plug on Alysa. We need prayer that it will never happen." She shared other events and concerns and then made two more phone calls, one to Grandma Rivers and another to Faith Baptist for the prayer chain. She thought to herself, those doctors are going to be in for a real surprise on Thursday when they find out what the power of prayer is all about.

The dreaded Thursday arrived. It was 8:45 a.m. on Day 186 of

171

Alysa's hospitalization. Ken, Sylvia, Linda and Lamar the EEG technician stood by while Dr. Baskin read the latest EEG. Her face was strained by the discouragement she felt.

Pastor Jim and Ray Thomas had come earlier to say hello, offer support and pray just outside the meeting while it was being conducted. The meeting started at 9:35. Present were Dr. Baskin, Dr. Landau, Shirley the social worker, Nurse Marilyn, Jerry Stephens and the Conselyea contingent. Dave nervously placed a tape recorder in the middle of the table. The meeting ended at 10:00. The life support issue had not been mentioned.

A fax had arrived in the night from Crooked Creek Convalescent Home in Grand Blanc that they had a placement for Alysa. The doctors discussed Alysa's dismissal instead.

"God provides for those who love him and are faithful! This placement is a result of prayer. I'm sure of it. Isn't it wonderful? He just took away the entire issue!" Linda excitedly announced.

"It's a good thing, too. If we had needed documentation, we were out of luck. I forgot to turn the tape recorder on," Dave admitted.

"Oh, Dave. You are too much," Linda said as she squeezed him in a bear hug.

He returned the hug with undaunted enthusiasm.

Additional good news was relayed to those who were faithful in prayer when Linda made the phone calls, "Besides the phenomenal timing of Lysa's acceptance by Crooked Creek, her blood clot dissolved. Thank you for your prayers!"

The children's song about the prayers going up and the blessings coming down kept playing in Linda's mind.

The day before her departure for the next leg of her journey, Alysa had company. Mike and Lisa McCulloch, Linda Two, Carrie, Kelly, Ken, Grandma and Grandpa Rivers, and of course Mom and Dad. Linda Two, Carrie and Kelly gave Alysa their now famous spa treatment a la hospital bed. With a facial, a hairdo, shaved legs and a pedicure, Alysa would wow them at her new home.

All the nurses came in to say their good-byes. They gave Alysa a card and a cross imbedded in a crystal casing.

The journal entry on Day 189, with 58 of those days spent at St. Vincent's Hospital, closed with, "We read and prayed with Alysa."

*   *   *   *   *

Any moving day causes apprehension, excitement and challenge. Moving from St. Vincent's to Crooked Creek, some 70 miles away, created its own set of circumstances. Logistics with transportation, carefully arranged, allowed one parent to ride in the ambulance while the other drove to Grand Blanc. A car had already been dropped off in Grand Blanc so Linda and Dave could both have a car available.

Thus, the morning started early for the Conselyeas. As they drove to St. Vincent's they chatted happily about the impending move and their hopes for Alysa.

"I am so glad that Alysa is leaving St. Vincent's. The doctors were so cold and callous to Alysa and to us, don't you think, Dave?" Linda asked, looking for agreement.

"You're right on, Honey. I know they were busy and had lots of patients, but that's no excuse for the way they treated us. It's like they didn't really believe she could get any better. To think that they wanted us to pull the plug. I still can't get over it."

"The nurses and the therapists were wonderful, though. I think nurses deserve all the credit. They do all the hard work. Plus, they truly care about the patient. I'm not surprised that so many are believers."

"I agree," Dave said. "Most of them were loving and caring. There are only a few in this whole ordeal that I didn't particularly care for."

They put this past experience behind them and looked only to the future. Arriving at the hospital, they parked the car and headed for Alysa's room. They were met by Shirley just outside Alysa's room.

"I'm afraid I have some bad news," she started.

Dave and Linda stopped dead in their tracks, frowns on their faces.

"The form for Alysa's Medicaid somehow didn't get sent in last week. It will be another week before the paperwork is finished and she can leave. I'm sorry."

"I just don't believe it," Dave said. "How could that happen? Isn't there some way around it? For crying out loud!"

"You know," Linda began, "It would have been nice if you

173

could have called us and told us. We now have a car up in Grand Blanc that we have to go pick up. A little consideration would have been appreciated."

That "week" turned into twenty-four days. During that time Linda was confronted again and again by the several doctors who were questioning her tenacious hold on the belief that her daughter would survive. On the other hand, just as many others encouraged Linda and girded her faith.

Kim Fuhrman, a mortgage rep that Dave knew, dropped in to see and pray with Alysa. Kim told of her brother who was in a serious auto accident and had survived. Not bothered by the suctioning and the network of tubes, she held Alysa's hand and talked to her.

"You are on my daily prayer list. God can heal you. Just trust in him. The doctors aren't always right," she told Alysa. Then to Linda, she said from her own experience, "Don't let Satan use the doctors to discourage you."

"That's exactly what I needed to hear. I had quite a confrontation with Jerry Stephens, one of the physician's assistants. He was angry with me for my not wanting to delay the trials to wean her off the respirator. Alysa had been extremely agitated and had definitely had seizure activity. We totally disagreed on her having CPAP treatments, or the breathing on her own. Our conversation was not pleasant, to say the least!

"Then I attended my leader's meeting with BSF and my feelings were soothed. I was again reminded that God was in control and that he was bigger than Jerry Stephens. If I remained faithful to my Bible study and to God, God would take care of Alysa. I replaced my anger with prayer as I drove back to the hospital. I encountered the P.A again, only this time I was prepared. The Holy Spirit helped the words flow from my lips.

"I explained that my trust was in God not in them, the doctors. I told him that God had a very special plan for Alysa and that his timing and his plan for her were perfect. The bottom line is that they didn't know how to 'fix' Alysa. For them it was a very difficult situation. If I had thought their doctors could fix my daughter, they'd have had to admit me to the psychiatric ward by now. How else could I have withstood the roller coaster ride that we'd been on?"

174

"What happened next?" Kim asked.

"Well, I imagine, by the look on Jerry's face, he thought I'd already gone around the bend. Then he asked me, 'If you trust in God, why don't you let her go back to her God?'"

"I'll tell you why, Jerry. I have already spent a lot of time over that very thought. I have taken that question to the Lord and each time I have not been given peace with the decision to let her go. I told him I wouldn't try to hang on any longer. Jerry again gave me his pessimistic opinion of her recovery. Then I really got wound up.

"Do you think I'm so selfish as a mother that I just want to see my daughter lie here day after day with all those tubes coming out all over her? God has told me that he will heal her and I believe that with all my heart and mind."

"Then what did he say?" Kim wanted to know.

"You know, I don't really remember. I guess he just heard me out and decided not to spar with such a Loony Toon. He didn't know what hit him."

Kim and Linda continued talking and Kim left a gift book for Alysa.

Friends of Alysa's came to visit. Jen Lucas had to step out and cry before she could even approach Alysa's bed. Katie Morgan was stronger and managed to keep up a cheerful chatter over Alysa's bedside. Linda considered it a blessing that they had not forgotten their friend. Jen was again in tears when she left.

"Thanks for coming," she told the two young women.

Linda was encouraged again one night when one of the fun-loving nurses was telling Alysa a funny traffic ticket story. Alysa seemed to respond by shaking her head, twice. They called the other nurses in to see for themselves. Excitement broke out.

Dr. Baskin was still on the scene and informed them that the other doctors were requesting that they sign a DNR, or Do Not Resuscitate, for the records in case Linda and Dave couldn't be reached. The Conselyeas remained firm in their conviction and their decision. N-O.

In the middle of the night Dave prayed that Alysa's temperature would go below 100 and stay there. God answered that prayer. Dave practically tapped everyone on the shoulder and said, "Do you know what God did? He lowered my daughter's temperature when I asked him to. What do you think of that?"

5:00 a.m. Hey, Ken, I beat you in. I couldn't sleep since I didn't see my little girl last night. I'm still in a state of awe that God would grant my prayer about Alysa's temp. It's not that I don't believe he could do it, it's just that lately I guess I've been afraid he wasn't listening. Thank you Lord! 5:15 I have the privilege of feeding Alysa this morning. Janet is nurse. She had Christmas music playing. 6:00 Breathing therapy in for treatment. She was a little low on blood ox (92). Suctioned and got lots of "goobers." B. O. rose to 99%. H.R.=102. Last temp=98.6. PTL. I don't know exactly when they did it but she has an IV back in. I guess her urine output was low. I gave her an extra syringe of water after breakfast. 6:30 Resp back in to take off treatment and suction some more. I called LRC to make sure she was up and at 'em. Listening to Manheim Steamroller. 3:30 LRC reading to Alysa. 4:05 Eyes turning to right. Some stiffness. Arms stiff. 40 minutes. 4:45 Resp treatment. Lungs clear after treatment. 5:00 I sat Alysa up. Started strong coughing at 6:00. Showing off—lifting head off bed. Raising arms. H.R.=108. Fed Alysa. 7:00 Clear eyes. 8:00 Dad here with chicken from Chicken Shack (Mom's favorite). Brought some for the nurses. Secretary said this floor is spoiled. 9:10 Alysa's temp is 99.5! Starting to move legs again. Mouth and fingers also moving. 10:15 Ken, Linda and I praying with Alysa after Bible reading. 11:15 Dr. Baskin in. Alysa responsive and moving right arm up to trache and moving legs. 11:30 Going home. Alysa sweating, seems upset. Calmed her down the best I could. Love you Sweetie Pie. God's watching over you.

Linda and Dave didn't always understand the behavior of the doctors. That night Dr. Baskin had made all of her chart notes outside the room.

"Why do you think she goes out of the room to write on the chart?" Ken asked.

"I'm baffled by her actions," Linda responded. "She's a young doctor, close to Alysa's age. Maybe she has her own fears of mortality. Who knows?"

"She seems a little standoffish to me," Dave said. "She is just one of those doctors who can't hold hands or get close to the patient. It's her loss."

As Murphy's Law has it, some satisfaction and explanation surfaced at the end of Alysa's St. Vincent's stay. Linda had the opportunity to discuss her daughter's case with the head neurologist when she requested recent copies of Alysa's EEG's and MRI's. He referred to Alysa as "Mystery Girl." He found her case baffling. It had too many facets to consider—the encephalitis, the Haldol, the non-normal seizure pattern, and of course, Alysa's inability to talk to shed any light on how she felt. Linda told him about the games being played between the pulmonology department and Dr. Baskin.

"As soon as Dr. Baskin wrote the order for a neuro drug, the pulmonologist would mark it out and write what he wanted," she said. "Alysa seemed to be the ping pong ball between the two departments. Also, they dragged their feet when it came to weaning her from the respirator."

The doctor lowered his glasses, made notations on a pad and became more interested in her account.

"I wish I had known," he said to Linda. "If you had given me the word, I would have fired the whole team and had a new team in the next day."

"I didn't know that we had that option. Hindsight is always 20-20. I also had many disturbing conversations with one of the physician's assistants. He said that neurology was only in charge of this much—the brain," she showed a half-inch between her thumb and first finger.

"And that the pulmonologists were in charge of this much— the entire body!" She spread her hands apart wide. "The P.A. challenged me on several occasions."

"That sounds like inexcusable behavior to me," Dr. Gratinelli said. " I'm so sorry that you were treated rudely. I can assure you that I will deal with that. On a different subject, I want to recommend neurologists in Grand Blanc. You will want the very best to handle your daughter's case."

Linda would have to change her blanket opinion of the doctors at St. Vincent's. There was at least one who was compassionate and kind. But again, it was not with the doctors that her trust lay.

CHAPTER FOURTEEN

On her ambulance ride from St. Vincent's to Crooked Creek, Alysa had her dad to keep her company this time. The two Lindas were still en route when the ambulance wheeled up to the entrance. They were met by Christa, Lysa's primary care nurse.

"Welcome, welcome," she said, greeting the pair at the door. "Hi, Alysa. Let's get you set up in your new room."

Once Alysa was settled, Christa iterated the upcoming events to Dave. "Your daughter will receive a whirlpool bath at least twice a week, we'll have her dressed and up in a chair every other day, and the staff will give her their very best attention. If you want to just stay here with Alysa and fill out these papers, I'll continue getting her comfortable."

Dave attacked the familiar paperwork with a lightness of heart. The nurse turned her attention and conversation to Alysa.

"First, Alysa, we're going to remove that catheter. Then...."

"Boy, you will have a friend for life," Dave interrupted. "She's hated that darn thing for 214 days!"

"Well, it's our policy that our patients not use a catheter. We will make sure that she is changed every two hours. She'll be kept dry."

As if to test the promise, Alysa chose that time to relieve her bladder and her bowels. She was cleaned up immediately. Alysa seemed alert and her eyes tracked Christa and all the people who

178

came in and out of her room that day.

The two Lindas arrived shortly after 10:00 a.m. They fussed around Alysa and her room arranging the boom box, the posters and cards, and stuffed animals. They had the room "homified" in minutes. Dave left for work mid-day, but returned by 7:00. Ken walked in just minutes after Dave.

"Say, there's a Christmas party down in the meeting room. The nurse told me we could go down and help ourselves," he announced.

"What are we waiting for?" asked Dave.

The two returned laden with Christmas cookies and other calorie-laced goodies.

"I just love Christmas," Dave gushed, munching on crackers with a cheese ball spread. "Here, girls, have some," he offered to Linda and Linda Two.

"You just go ahead and pig out. We're ready to head back to Royal Oak. How long do you think you'll stay?"

"Oh, probably till eleven or so. I should be home around midnight."

"I'll be asleep," Linda said offering her cheek for a kiss.

Dave grabbed her, saying, "You don't get off that easy." He hugged and kissed his wife good night.

Don, the night nurse, came in to feed Alysa. Dave watched his technique with the bolis feeding because it matched his own.

"Hey, I like you already," he said to the nurse. "You're careful to adjust the syringe into the tube and you pour the food slowly." Dave observed and noted how the canned nutrition went into Alysa's feeding tube, helped only by gravity. He approved. "Sometimes a nurse will feed her too quickly and then she gets sick."

While the nighttime quiet crept room by room throughout the convalescent center, Dave approached his daughter and gently lifted her hand to his lips. "I love you," he whispered. He read Psalm 91 and then bowed his head to pray. With the transfer to Crooked Creek, a new chapter in her life had begun.

Alysa was sitting in the lounge in a recliner chair next to the nurses' station when Linda arrived the next day. "My, aren't we getting spoiled right away?" She took a seat next to her and started reading aloud another section from *The Power of Prayer.*

Linda contemplated her new situation. She felt pretty isolated and alone. The Grand Blanc location now separated her from her support group: her parents, Linda Two and her daughters, Carrie and Kelly, Ken, and her sister, Carol. Even Dave was unable to come more than once a day. The advantage of the move was that she and Dave could return to their own home and have a life together after living with her parents for seven months. Her reverie halted when one of the cheery aides sat down beside her.

"We want you to consider Crooked Creek Alysa's home. The entire building is at your disposal. Bring in a Christmas tree if you want to. Feel free to push her recliner chair to the lobby, to the meeting room—anywhere you want to go. In fact, Happy Hour is at 3:00. Honey Lee sings and plays the piano and there will be light refreshments. Just let any of us know if you need anything, okay?"

"Thank you so much. I was feeling a bit overwhelmed by the newness and you have made me feel much better. Bless you!"

Happy Hour frightened Alysa. She scrunched her eyes, tensed her body and pulled her head and shoulders up as if she were saying, "Get me out of here!" They left as Honey Lee finished "Beer Barrel Polka" and started "Let Me Call You Sweetheart." Alysa's age was one-fourth that of most of the residents'age. But it was the noise and different surroundings that had alarmed her, not the choice of musical pieces.

I do think she'll love her whirlpool bath, Linda told herself, focusing on something positive.

Breathing treatments by the respiratory staff and the physical therapy arm and leg manipulation were conducted in the same manner as before in the hospital. Suctioning the trache was old hat and the bolis feedings were not new. So all Alysa had to adjust to were a new location and unfamiliar faces. She continued to run fevers, to have non-functional arm and hand movement, to sweat, and to be non-responsive to her environment. And she was still dependent on life support.

On Monday, December 16, Linda drove to Ortonville to see Stuart, a decorator friend, and to pick up a wall hanging Christmas tree for Alysa's room. Stuart was fond of Alysa and was happy to do something for her.

"Oh, Stuart! This tree is magnificent. You did a beautiful job.

How much do I owe you?"

"Absolutely nothing. Nada," he protested.

"But I intend to pay you for it."

"No way! I wish I could do more for you and Alysa. This is such a tiny token of what I want to do. If it brings her pleasure, that's all I want."

"I can't tell you how much I appreciate this. I'll be sure to emphasize to Alysa that this is from you. It's going to be a hard Christmas, not having Lysa home with us. Putting this gorgeous tree up in her room at Crooked Creek is going to buoy our festive attitudes. I'm just overwhelmed."

"Don't be. Just tell her Merry Christmas from me. And to get well soon!"

Linda left the shop in better spirits thinking of the generosity of her friend. As she drove to Grand Blanc, a beautiful snowfall had begun to coat the gray surroundings, transforming them into a winter spectacle. The fat, fluffy flakes fell so furiously that the windshield wipers couldn't keep up the pace. Linda, her parka covered with snow, tramped into Alysa's room with the tree protected in a large bag. She shed her coat onto the floor with her eagerness to present the tree.

"Look, Alysa, Stuart Smith made this for you," she said, holding it up in front of Alysa. "Let's plug it in over here so you can see it from your bed." She moved a chair out of the way, removed a picture from the wall and stood on her tiptoes to fasten the tree to the picture hanger. "There! Now, let's plug it in." The lights sparkled and the ambiance of the entire room changed in a second. It was Christmas. Within moments, the news spread and the staff and even some patients came in to see it. Linda knew that it was the envy of the whole facility.

A slew of visitors queued up at Alysa's bedside her first week at Crooked Creek. Grandma and Grandpa Conselyea visited on Saturday. Nikki came with Ken on Sunday, Pat, Christy and Becky Toth visited Monday, Sandy Barnes and Marilyn Wisner came Wednesday. On Thursday, Lisa Freese Hine, Jennifer Dowey Stricker and Ethel Freese came with a beautiful potted purple mum. Lisa and Alysa had been college roommates. The three visitors cried when they comprehended the extent of Alysa's situation. Grandma and Grandpa Rivers visited on the weekend.

Mark Biddle, one of the respiratory therapists from Oakhill Memorial, drove up to see Alysa. He had stayed in touch throughout her entire illness. He brightened upon seeing Alysa sitting in her recliner chair in the lobby, or living room, as Linda deemed it. It was Alysa's Tuesday visitor who surprised Linda.

Andrea Cox McCracken walked two miles in the snow from her apartment in Grand Blanc to see her friend. She was in the middle of telling Alysa about a mutual friend's wedding when Linda came into the room.

"Oh, and it was so funny. Dennis was so nervous while he waited for Wendy to come down the aisle. You could see the sweat on his face. When he saw Wendy, he looked like he was going to pass out. She was cool. Her dress was just awesome. I think it had been her mother's and it had some beading added to it. The reception was at...oh, hi, Mrs. Conselyea."

"Hi, Andrea. It's so good to see you! How are you?" she asked, hugging her daughter's friend from high school.

"I'm just fine. I was telling Lysa about Wendy's wedding. Everyone wanted to know how she was doing."

Andrea stayed most of the day. She related who of their married friends was pregnant and who wanted to be and all the other girl topics that held fascination. She helped Linda give Alysa a shampoo and bath.

Around 5:00 she asked, "Do you suppose you could give me a ride home, Mrs. Conselyea!"

"Well, of course I could. How did you get here?"

"I walked."

"In the snow?"

"It didn't seem that far. It was so pretty. I actually enjoyed it."

In the car, Andrea, a Christian and graduate of Bob Jones University, turned to Linda and said, "I don't know how you can stand this illness and the way Alysa is. How in the world have you managed? What has kept you from totally losing it?"

It seemed strange for Linda to share the strength of her faith with someone who already knew the Lord. "God has told us that he will never forsake us and it's true. He is there with Alysa in her room. He is here with us in the car. He is my rock, my strength and my encouragement. Without the knowledge of his promises, I would fall apart. He's my glue. He is going to heal her. He told me he would."

"Wow! That's so neat. I hope my faith grows to be as strong as yours." She didn't realize she was making a prophetic statement.

"Oh, it will, Honey." They pulled up to Andrea's apartment entrance. She had been motioning the directions while Linda was driving. "Thank you for coming to see Lysa. It means more than you can imagine."

Surprise visitors that evening were especially welcome. Mary Kay, one of the third shift nurses, brought her son and his Boy Scout troop to sing carols to the residents. They went room to room and serenaded each person. Some performed seriously with great intent and others gawked, jostled and sang off key. It so touched Linda that she had to turn her head so they wouldn't see her tears. Memories filled her mind of Alysa and her dancing class going to entertain at nursing homes nine or ten years earlier. She remembered the enthusiasm of the girls in their cute little costumes and the pleasure in the eyes of the audience. She never thought Alysa would be lying in a bed listening to the voices of nine uniformed 10-year-old boys with yellow kerchiefs tied around their necks. She was deeply moved.

Bedecked with another decorated Christmas tree, Ken strode into the room. Kristin, a friend of Carrie's that Linda hadn't met, and other friends of Alysa's wanted her to know that they were thinking of their friend. Ken placed it so all four of the women in the room—Alysa and her three roommates—could enjoy it.

Wednesday, December 18
Day 220

9:15 Dad here. Boy does my girl look good. Christa is in and Doctor McCaffrey to see Alysa. Everybody loves the decorations. The room looks beautiful. 9:30 Nurses aides here. Going to give Alysa a whirlpool. I told her how much she is going to enjoy it. 9:45 Lanie from Resp in to suction. I just did it. 10:00 I'm down in lounge having a Diet Coke and waiting for the whirlpool to be over. P.S. To Alysa. Ken spent the night in your room last night. That's a first. And to think he even had our permission. 10:30 Lanie says Alysa was swimming. 10:40 I'm with Alysa and she looks neat. She's got her blue shorts and halter top on with her white Mickey Mouse tennis shoes. We are sitting outside her room. She's in her special reclining chair. She seems comfortable. Temp-101.2. Christa getting Tylenol. I will feed her lunch. 11:00 Resp therapist got blood ox reading=93%. Pulse=97. She's not unhappy with that. A young lady from McCaffrey's office came out and gave me a comfortable office chair to sit in. Everyone keeps coming down to check on us. 1:00 Linda here now. I'm leaving for the office. I love you, Sweetie.

Alysa had spoken few intelligible words since May 17, 1996. Her response to stimulation consisted of occasional mumbling and slight body movements. But it was Christmas and spirits were festive.

*   *   *   *   *

Ken attended church the Sunday before Christmas with Alysa's parents. It felt strange and sad not to have Alysa sitting in the pew with them. They chose the Duck Blind restaurant in Waterford for brunch afterwards. They shared their plans for the day.

"So, you're going to Crooked Creek now?" Dave asked Ken.

"Yeah. I'll be there all day. What about you guys?"

"Well, since you're going to be there, I think we'll head down to Livonia and pay our respects to Poncho's family at the funeral home. We should get to Grand Blanc early this evening."

"Man, that was really tragic. A senseless death. Do they know who shot him?"

"No, just a whacko delivery guy, I guess. Judy, Poncho's wife, can identify him so I hear she's under police protection. She was shot, too, but only wounded. Poncho and I were Kareoke buddies. We met the Gonzales at a party at a friend's house in the early Eighties," Dave said. "I still can't believe he's gone."

"You can reach us on the car phone if you need us for any reason," Linda said. "Give Lys a kiss for us," she added.

"No problem." Ken smiled.

Their cars exited the gray slushy parking lot and headed in different directions.

Ken listened to the radio on his northbound drive. Traditional carols and lively Christmas music played. "I'll Be Home For

Christmas" began and he quickly punched the station selector. Maybe next year, he desperately hoped.

He found Alysa in the hallway sitting in her recliner. She seemed to be in distress. She was hot, sweaty and tense, and her arm made jerking motions from the armrest into the air.

"Hi, Babe," he said giving her a kiss on the forehead.

"That's from your parents. Now here's mine," and he kissed her again on the mouth.

Next he felt her forehead. "You're burning up." He left in search for the nurse.

At the nurse's station he inquired, "Who's on for Alysa today?"

"I am," Travis said. "What do you need?"

"What's her temp? She feels pretty warm to me."

"I know. She had a whirlpool this morning, and loved it, I might add. But her fever has been rising all day. I've called the doctor about it."

Satisfied that the staff was on top of the situation, Ken returned to be with Alysa. By late afternoon, her temperature spiked to 105. Travis told Ken the doctor's orders.

"She has to be admitted to the hospital. There could be infection or pneumonia. We're sending her to St. Mary's."

Ken tried to reach the Conselyeas. He hung up when he heard, "The cellular number you are calling is turned off or out of the service area. Please try your call later." So he called his mother instead.

"Hi, Mom. I couldn't reach Dave on his car phone. Alysa has a high fever and is being taken to St. Mary's here in Grand Blanc. Would you call Mrs. Rivers and between the two of you, maybe you can reach Dave and Linda?"

"Sure. Are there any other problems?"

"I don't know. It could be infection or pneumonia."

Dave and Linda stopped at home at 6:00 to finally change out of their church clothes. They discussed the kindness of Poncho's close-knit family at the funeral home.

"To think that Eddie, in all the pain of losing his father, asked how Alysa was doing. That just blows my mind," Dave said.

"But," Linda said, "God lets people suffer so they can better understand and help others who are suffering. There's an understanding empathy that only the Lord can create. We truly can feel each other's pain."

"Yeah, not like you-know-who."

"You mean Slick Willie? Oh, Dave, would you get the phone? I'm going into the bathroom."

"Dave. Sylvia. I sure wish you would get a working answering machine. Ken called. Alysa has spiked a high fever and she was being taken to St. Mary's in Grand Blanc."

"Oh, Lord!"

"Call me when you find out how she is."

"Okay, Mom. We will."

Dave rapped on the bathroom door. "Linda! Hurry up. We've got to go."

"What's wrong? Who was on the phone?"

"It was your mom. Lysa's got a high fever and is being hospitalized."

"Oh, Dave. Not for Christmas!"

They tore out of the house to face the new emergency. They arrived at St. Mary's only to learn that Alysa had been rerouted to Mid Town Hospital because St. Mary's CAT scan was not in service.

After being lost, twice, they entered Mid Town's emergency room. Alysa's temperature had been successfully lowered, but the cause had not been identified. The high fever had initiated seizure movements and had put Alysa into a hyperactive state.

When Linda witnessed the reappearance of the dreaded movements, she experienced a physical blow. She stepped out of the room. With her eyes tightly shut and her body shaking with pain she whispered, "Lord, I can't deal with this. Please, please help me."

Within seconds of her beseeching request, in walked Tom and Brenda Cox, friends to support and console her. Steve Moffett also showed up after a circuitous trip from Crooked Creek to St. Mary's to Mid Town. They rallied round Linda, Dave and Ken and prayed for the emergency at hand.

Shortly after midnight, Alysa was admitted to ICU room number 602. Dr. Wickenberg from the Pulmonary Department spoke to the parents.

"I'd like to get some detailed information from you folks if you're not too tired. Your daughter's medical records have accompanied her, but it looks like it would take me a week to plow through them."

"That's for sure. I'm Dave Conselyea and this is my wife, Linda."

They shook hands and the doctor led them to an empty conference room nearby. He asked probing questions and listened attentively to their answers. The East Lansing "something bad happened" resurfaced, but this time Dave could discount it. He had received a documented time line from the very cooperative Redken representative he had contacted. It accounted for every moment of Alysa's weekend and ruled out a physical assault.

With apparent compassion, the doctor conversed, unhurriedly, for forty-five minutes. He concluded with an assessment. "I think we need a neurologist here to see Alysa right away. I'm going to see if I can get Dr. Broadmoor to come in. He's the best."

Dr. Wickenberg's opinion of Dr. Broadmoor was off the mark. He was better than the best, Linda later would state.

"He is one of the nicest doctors we have encountered," she told Dave with feeling. "He is recommending the special 24-hour EEG for Alysa at Jerry Rush Hospital, and he is the one with the pull to arrange it. I'm just thrilled!"

Dave rubbed his chin and responded, "Maybe that's why Alysa contracted pneumonia. To get her in here so she could connect with Dr. Broadmoor. God has put her in the right place at the right time with the right people. It's awesome."

"You're right. It's all in his timing. Speaking of which, Alysa has to recover from her current infection before she can have the test, but Dr. Broadmoor says he won't forget us."

Although none of the Conselyeas looked forward to celebrating Christmas in the hospital, the situation was made easier by their acceptance that God was in control—still.

The Conselyeas tried to muster brave facades, but their Christmas Eve lacked its festive luster. It would have been a complete bomb if the Toths hadn't shown up. Leaving for England on Christmas Day didn't deter their visit.

"I can't think of anyone who would have Christmas Eve dinner in a hospital cafeteria on purpose," Linda said.

"Especially when they're leaving for London the next day,"

187

Dave added.

"Well, our refrigerator was empty. And Christmas is in the heart, not the stomach, right?" said Pat.

"I'm not too sure. This dressing and gravy is much better than yours," Pete said, which earned him an elbow in the side. "Oomph. Okay, I'll retract that!"

Christy and Becky eagerly talked of their upcoming itinerary. Their youthful enthusiasm combined with the bedside attention Pete and Pat gave Alysa made for a joyful occasion after all.

"Thank God for friends," said Linda as she hugged them good-bye.

"Hey, do you say 'Bon Voyage' when you're flying or is that just for ships?" Dave wanted to know. "Thanks for coming by."

"And thanks for the cookies. Merry Christmas!" Linda said.

"Merry Christmas."

Those two words echoed in their ears. Yes, Christmas exists in the heart.

Ken, his sisters Kelly and Carrie, and Tom, Carrie's boyfriend, came to see Alysa on Christmas Day. It helped Linda and Dave to get through the day. After the visitors left, they opened their gifts.

"I think Alysa likes her gifts, don't you?" he asked Linda.

He had held up each gift for Alysa's unseeing eyes and had conjured enough response for both of them. He perceived that she liked them.

Yeah, she liked them, he told himself.

Linda washed Alysa's hair and fed her dinner through the stomach tube. Both doctors came in on Christmas to check on their patient. Linda was touched.

Steve Moffett returned, the second time in four days, to be with his longtime friend. Dave read the Christmas story from the chapter of Luke. At least that family tradition remained unchanged.

At 9:40 Alysa received a hospital Christmas present: she was moved out of ICU to a private room on a medical floor. Linda prayed with her daughter, kissed her good night, and bade Dave and Steve farewell. Steve had volunteered to drop Dave off on his way home. At midnight, after prayer, Dave kissed his daughter good-bye.

"Good night, Sweetheart. Merry Christmas."

*   *   *   *   *

Linda was on the phone with Dave. "The vampires are gone," she told him.

"They are? What happened?"

Vampires was their pet name for all of the nurses and doctors who stuck Alysa every day to either draw blood or deliver medications. Alysa's body, covered with scar tissue, had no veins remaining for entry.

"I signed for Dr. King to do a small surgery to put a semi-permanent line in her right arm. It's called a pass-port. It is considered invasive surgery. A line or small tube is inserted in the vein and goes to the heart. A small sponge-like opening, located just beneath the skin, seals itself when it is not is use. It allows for the quick administering of drugs in an emergency. She can get her daily antibiotics and drugs through it. No more probing and searching for a vein. Dr. King told me that sometimes they last three to five years. He sure was nice."

"I hope Lysa doesn't have need for it that long," Dave said.

The pass-port was one of the good things that happened. Alysa spent the holiday season with open, unfocused eyes. She had periods of seizure movements, grinding of teeth, profuse sweating, intense suctioning, rigid muscles and overall discomfort. Her lips moved, her eyes blinked, her tongue stuck out, and she patted her chest with her hands. Three new medications were introduced: Zantac to prevent stomach ulcers, Claform for infection and Clindemycin for pneumonia. She had BM's and was cleaned up. Vomit and cleaned up. Saliva, secretions, and sweat and cleaned up. "And a partridge in a pear tree."

*   *   *   *   *

Alysa was back home at Crooked Creek for New Year's Eve. The transfer lessened Linda's stress. She came in to wash her daughter's hair so she would look good for her date with Ken. He arrived at 6:00 so Dave and Linda could attend a New Year's Eve party.

At 11:00, Ken removed Alysa's protective booties and gave her a thorough foot massage. He exhibited his thoughts, feelings and desires in his slow, loving movements. Jay Leno provided the backdrop for their date. As 1996 gave way to 1997, Ken toasted his Sweetheart.

"Happy New Year! Here's to a great New Year," he said as he tenderly kissed Alysa's lips.

"I love you."

Just outside the door, a nurse observed his affectionate display. She gulped down her sudden rush of emotion and ran to hide her unbidden tears. I hope they have a great New Year, she fervently wished. Please God.

Interview with Pat Toth

A wrought iron teapot stand in the front yard. A teapot on the front door. Teapots on every shelf and cabinet. Teapots on the breakfront. Teapots in the windowsill. Teapots on the piano. Pat Toth and teapots are synonymous. She started collecting her more than 50 teapots a few years ago, and sort of got carried away. Except for her affinity for teapots and tea parties, Pat Toth is as normal as anyone else. Pat was a frequent visitor during Alysa's hospitalization and was one of Linda's prayer partners.

Pat tells about herself and her visits:

Linda and I were in the same discussion group in Bible Study Fellowship. Eager to discuss the lessons, we got in the habit of going out to lunch after each study. Linda's love for the Lord is so evident, and she likes to talk about what he's done for her. God has done so much in my own life.

I was saved when I was 17. I had not been raised in a Christian home. Three days after high school graduation, I took off and flew to California. I landed eventually in Balboa Park in San Diego where the "Jesus Freaks" were. These were the Seventies and the "find yourself" generation. I was searching—a little curious— hostile to their message, but I hung around anyway. I was definitely not interested in the gospel of John tract that Burt, one of the "Freaks" handed out. In a bored, lonely moment weeks later, I picked up the tract, read it, and accepted Christ into my life. I returned to Balboa Park to find Burt and tell him, but they had moved on. I'll see Burt in heaven and I'll tell him then.

It took two years for that acceptance to grow into complete understanding. I floundered until God sent the right person to teach and minister to me. That's why I now feel so strongly about disciplining new Christians in the church. I met Pete in San Diego and we were baptized before we were married. We were hungry for the Word and attended every class and seminar we could find. God has planned our lives from the beginning and will until the very end.

I first learned of Alysa's illness at BSF when we were asked to pray for her. She was in the hospital and seemed to be hallucinating and suffering from a psychological problem. My husband, Pete, and other deacons from the church went to pray for her. Pete came home and said that Dave was coming apart. He had been talking to Alysa, and she just stopped talking. Now her tongue was hanging out and she was non-responsive.

When I first saw Alysa, I was shocked. Seeing her completely incapacitated and incoherent contrasted starkly with the perfectly healthy young girl she was only days before. To think that it could be my own child brought reality crashing down around me. It made me value my own children. On days thereafter when I thought I was having a bad or stressful day, I'd forget the pity party and just think of Linda at the hospital sitting next to her comatose daughter for 10 to 12 hours at a time. I hoped I could be an encourager to Linda.

I could usually hear the Christian music playing before I entered Alysa's hospital room. I'd greet her, tell her who I was and talk to her as if she were awake. Hi, I'm Pat Toth, your mother's friend, and this is my husband, Pete. Linda had stressed to everyone that doctors believe that coma patients can hear and process much of what they hear, so to never talk discouragingly about or to Alysa. So we were always very careful to talk positively to Alysa and not about her.

Often I took my teenage daughters, Christy and Becky, along. We would mention names of her friends from Springfield Christian Academy. We'd tell her that Roy, Jennifer, Tara and Ondrea all say Hi, and that at least 50 people at church had asked about her. I was reading in the Psalms today that God will hold you in his hands I would mention. And always, we prayed aloud for her.

When she was in ICU, I'm afraid we lied. Only family is allowed into ICU to see the patients. We said that we were family so we could see her. Well, we are all in the family of God, aren't we? I vividly remember one of those times. Alysa seemed to be choking. She was having trouble breathing. The nurses tended to her and suctioned out the secretions that were hindering her breathing. To me, it was alarming. To Linda, it was routine. To me, it was the "crash team." To Linda it was another day. My heart went out to Linda that day. We became prayer partners.

Linda would call me each day and tell me what was going on. The prayer requests would be very specific. Pray that Alysa sleeps tonight. Pray that she opens her eyes. Pray that she learns to swallow. Pray for the infection in her trache neck opening. Pray that she has no more reaction to a drug. Each day had new prayer concerns. We prayed for weeks for Alysa to learn how to cough so she could get off the ventilator.

Linda would tell me how the Holy Spirit was working in their lives and in the lives of the people at the hospital. She wanted to know my prayer concerns for my own family. Linda was always very much aware of her purpose in ministering to others. Her focus was not entirely on herself and her problem. She sincerely cared about what others were experiencing. Every nurse, roommate and employee who came into the room heard about the Lord from Linda. We would visit Alysa thinking we were the encouragers and come away feeling buoyed and encouraged by Linda.

Her faith was steadfast. She never wavered or lost hope. Alysa had been moved to rehab and had started to show some progress. Then she started seizing continuously and was readmitted to St. Vincent's Hospital. It was a life-threatening situation. She was back on life support, back on the ventilator and in a deep, induced coma. That was a discouragingly dark time to me. I had faith that God could lift her up and heal her, but I didn't think he would. In my flesh, I gave up. It's a good thing that God didn't.

Until I met him at the hospital I hadn't known Dave other than to hear him sing in church. His devotion to Alysa was apparent. He spoke to Alysa so tenderly as he'd stroke her hand and face. He looked exhausted from his unselfish vigil at her bedside. He didn't know how their money situation would work out, but at first felt like he couldn't leave her to go to work.

When Alysa would thrash around, he needed to be there to protect her. After Alysa had been in so many facilities, he believed they couldn't leave her because they were the only two who knew what was going on.

Pete and Alysa had bonded when she was in the hospital. Men aren't always good around a sick person. Used to doing, they find inactivity difficult. One nice summer day, Linda and I had gone outside for a walk. Pete and the girls were watching Alysa. We had left Alysa on the floor on a sheet. When we returned, Alysa was sitting up in a chair. She had crawled crab-like across the floor and Pete had helped her to the chair. He didn't know that she had never done that before.

I have happier memories after Alysa entered the nursing home in Grand Blanc. Actually, the medical staff thought that would be merely a waiting ground for Alysa where she would simply vegetate. They were in for a surprise.

CHAPTER FIFTEEN

Monday, January 6, 1997
Day 239

11:30 p.m. I, Dave, am sitting here with Alysa and thanking God for her. I'm realizing that I have actually spent more quiet time and quality time with her since we've been in the hospital than all the years we've been together living under the same roof. It's sad, really, that it takes something this tragic to open my eyes to how much I love my family.

As I recall these past eight months and see how many people have taken Alysa into their prayer life, it really touches my heart. It may seem odd to give thanks to God for what seems to be an awful thing. I can't stop thinking how this sweet, wonderful young lady has caused so many people to come together with one purpose.

Alysa, I know that God is healing you and I know that you are coming back to Mom, Ken and me—your family and loved ones. You will be 100% recovered. Thank you, Sweetheart, for being the best daughter a dad could ever ask for. Good night, Sweetie. I love you.

The winter of 1997 matched the feelings and experiences of the Conselyeas. Their spirits rose high like a brisk sunshiny day only to be dashed like a bitter, road-blocking snowfall. The disappointing sameness of many days paralleled the day after day of gloomy winter weather. Hope and springtime—both seemed a long way off.

Alysa appeared to focus and tried to speak. Her trache was capped so speaking was possible. She was put on oxygen and breathed without the ventilator for four hours the first time, and on January 19, the vent was removed from the room. Alysa became more animated. She laughed, cried and gave her mother a kiss. She learned to hold her upper body upright and to keep her head from flopping side to side. Each offered an incremental step to be celebrated.

Super Bowl parties crowded the social calendar, and Dave and Linda did not want Alysa to be deprived. Their party was taken to Crooked Creek. Linda provided half the food: New England Clam Chowder and Wisconsin Cheese soup in honor of the two teams, the New England Patriots and the Green Bay Packers. Grandma Rivers brought shrimp, subs and chips. They prepared enough for the staff to join the festivities. Grandma and Grandpa Conselyea had visited earlier in the day, so they missed the party.

Alysa, surrounded by her family, was escorted to the conference room for her Super Bowl party. The big surprise was the arrival of Heidi, Alysa's little schnauzer. Her expected reaction to the beloved pet was deflating: Alysa appeared indifferent. Andy tried to reach his granddaughter another way.

"Lysa, your Aunt Dot from North Carolina called today to see how you're doing. We were talking about how much fun we all had when your grandma and I picked you up at Bob Jones University after your freshman year. Your cousins all say 'Hey!'

"Do you remember your first trip to North Carolina with us? We went to Cherokee and while there, you became fascinated by the Indian souvenirs and artifacts. I even found that photo of you with the feathered headdress the other day. Look, I brought it to show you. You loved the dancing. I think you wore your moccasins and danced around the house for a month. I want you to be dancing again, soon, you hear? I sure do."

Heads were nodding in agreement with Andy as he spoke— except Alysa's.

Ken and his mother arrived, and he gave Alysa a Michigan State nightshirt. Blankets and pillows had been put on the floor to see if Alysa preferred more freedom of movement. She didn't move around or explore the new territory. The staff loved the food and all in all, the party was a success, "especially since Green Bay won," Dave privately assessed.

Those who loved Alysa based their hope on miniscule improvements. Ken had one such moment when Lysa had been teasing him. He had tried to give her a kiss but she playfully pulled away. She turned away two or three times. When he offered his lips for another kiss, she moved toward him and really kissed back. But then she looked at him and cried. What pain or misery or failure of communication must she be suffering, Ken wondered.

Alysa was given a fenestrated trache—one that would allow sound to be transmitted without physical effort. Perhaps she had pent-up sounds because that evening her screams brought the entire staff to her room with her new capacity for emitting noise.

"I can't believe how alert and focused she seems," Linda said.

"I agree, but this screaming is too much," Dave replied.

Then Alysa clearly said, "No don't," followed by mumbled words. She kept that up until 1:30 a.m. After she finally calmed down, the Conselyeas prayed and went home.

Linda decided Alysa needed socialization and should attend Happy Hour again. She pushed Alysa's recliner past the nurses' station on the way to the Activities room. As she walked by she noticed the respiratory therapists in deep discussion. One of them called her aside.

"Linda, could we talk to you a minute? You know that soothing music you play in Alysa's room all the time?"

"Yes, the healing tape."

"What exactly is that?"

"Well, it's Christian Praise and Worship music. What about it?"

"All of the women in Alysa's room are showing great improvement. That's not the case in any of the other rooms. We think it is helping," she concluded.

Good observation, Linda thought. She said, "I'm glad that it is. Of course, there is a lot of prayer being offered in that room, too. Don't discount that."

Alysa was not enamored with Happy Hour—again.

The female residents at the nursing home planned to decorate sugar cookies for the Valentine's Day party. On February 12, Dave brought the decorations and toppings for the cookies that Linda provided. Linda checked to see how the decorating was going when she came in that afternoon.

Some women had use of only one hand or maybe a few fingers, and others could use both hands. A few just ate the frosting. But all of them were having a good time. They eagerly anticipated their Valentine's Ball. Local hair salons were donating time to fix hair, apply make up and give manicures. Volunteers even were bringing in formerly worn prom dresses for the women to wear.

That evening Alysa became beet red and her temperature soared to 105.4. The staff and Linda applied ice and towels to lower her fever. The fever had its dreaded effect: it set off seizure activity. Ken, Linda and the visiting Laneen hovered over Alysa's bed and prayed for her recovery. At 12:15 a.m., her twitching lessened and her fever broke. Dave stayed. The others went home.

Linda came in Valentine's Day to check on Alysa before leaving on her first trip away since Lys became ill. "Good morning, Sugar. Happy Valentine's Day. I'm going to Indianapolis for the weekend to see Cindy and John. Ken, Linda Two and Grandma are going to be here with you, okay? But before I leave, I want to take you down the hall. You really must see the women in their prom dresses. Let's go."

She pushed Alysa out into the hallway where the cosmetically enhanced, newly coifed women attired in prom dress finery sat in their wheelchairs awaiting the afternoon's ball. Alysa was dressed in red for the occasion, but her eveningwear was pajamas.

"Aren't they cute, Alysa? Hello, Mrs. Johnson. You look lovely today," she told one of the women. She handed out compliments as they walked down the hall. It is both wonderful and sad at the same time she thought. "Oh look, there's Grandma and Grandpa. Hi, Mom."

"Hi, Honey. Where should I put these tarts and pastries?"

Alysa's family always got involved with the people where Alysa was confined. Grandma Rivers had made enough Valentine goodies for three parties.

"I've got my Polaroid," Grandpa Rivers said, pointing to his gear. "These beautiful women need to be recorded for posterity."

The partygoers gloated in the attention they received from this kind man. The snapshots he later tacked on the bulletin board created conversation for many days. In Linda's absence Ken became the main caretaker. He encountered a non-responsive girlfriend who gazed at the ceiling with her mouth open, lips twitching, and hands fluttering. He dealt with high fevers, continuous suctioning of secretions, and runny bowel movements. He prayed with his Valentine before telling her good night.

Dave had resumed a fairly normal workday schedule and came to the nursing home in the evenings. When he thought that Linda needed some time to herself or some extra time in the mornings, he would try to see Alysa early in the morning. Often he'd stay longer than intended so he could oversee Alysa's care. The only activity that Linda kept was her Bible Study Fellowship meeting. Occasionally she would slip out for a quick lunch with friends, but primarily, she stayed at Alysa's bedside. The Conselyea's social life failed to exist. On rare evenings, Linda and Dave would attend an 11:00 p.m. movie in Flint just to have a few minutes together and to escape the realism of their ever-present vigil. Linda's weekend away felt like a sweepstakes vacation.

When Linda returned from her weekend in Indiana, Ken had several concerns he wanted to discuss with her. Linda, anxious for what she missed, asked for the details.

"Well," Ken began, "it could have been much worse. She was pretty uncomfortable the entire time, but nothing major happened. The nurses found congestion in her lungs and 'streaking' in her x-ray. She was absolutely full of gunk, so the suctioning was constant."

"What about her fever?"

"It didn't go away or spike, either. But the itching and scratching were—and still are—terrible. She just digs at herself, at her stomach and the, uh, 'baseball' scratch. Do you think we could cut her thumbnails? They seem to be doing the most damage. I didn't want to do it without asking. I know how you women are about your long nails."

Swallowing a smile, Linda said, "I think that's a good idea. We'll do it today."

"How was your visit? The Schmidlers?"

"The visit was really nice—the trip was the usual airline disaster: uncomfortable, crowded, no food and my flight home was delayed. But it was so good to see Cindy and John again. I met some of the people who have been praying for Alysa. That was an humbling experience to learn of their daily dedication to pray for someone they would never meet this side of heaven."

Interview with Cindy Schmidler

The rusty, slightly-drawled voice of Cindy Schmidler is housed in a slender, willowy frame. Earnest, big, hazel-green eyes peer from a cascade of blonde hair. Her love of the Lord punctuates her everyday conversation. It is no surprise that she and Linda are best friends.

Cindy tells about their friendship:

We met at Faith Baptist Church and coincidentally at Linda's Chocolate Cabbage Shop in Clarkston. But it was being together in Bible Study Fellowship that we really got to know each other. We would drive together and share how God was working in our lives.

Linda is warm, easy to know and exudes total unconditional love. I believe in all my heart that God brings people together, and he knew that I needed a good friend in Michigan. Our relocation to Michigan had been traumatic for me. I loved living in Indianapolis. We were content in a church. I had so many friends. I was in my comfort zone. But I didn't realize that I was stagnant in my growth with the Lord. Then, zap! We were in the Detroit area. John was working 24 hours a day with his new job, or so it seemed. We had lost our son, Jonathon, five days after his birth just a month before and we had a newly adopted infant son. I was miserable. Each day I was on my knees with the Lord, crying, why Lord? Why have you sent me here? Our perfect marriage was falling apart, I had no friends and it was cold!

Then I saw the light. I think the Holy Spirit shows us the way through prayer and the Word. I saw that I needed to change my attitude. God told me to grow up. He told me to get out of his way and let him take over. He was sovereign and was in control of my life. I changed profoundly and I stepped out in faith, but first I had suffered.

Linda and I were kindred spirits from past sufferings. We had both faced cancer. John and I were newly married when I was diagnosed with Hodgkin's disease. When I realized that I could die, I wanted to know about heaven. Our dear pastor, Dennis Fulton, came to our apartment weekly and held my hand and read scripture. We weren't even Christians yet, but we had a yearning for the truth. After I recovered, we both accepted Jesus as our Savior and had a personal relationship with our Lord.

With my new attitude, my life in Michigan changed and I grew spiritually. Pastor Jim's messages from the pulpit touched my heart and encouraged and challenged me. I was in the Word and had made new Christian friends from church and from Bible study. Any time that Linda, Dave, John and I were together, our focus was on the Lord and his love for us. Those outside of Christ can never fathom the comfort and joy of Christian fellowship. Dinners and after-church brunches with the Conselyeas and Alysa were always fun, and we admired the evident love between daughter and parents. Alysa's ready smile, her sense of humor and her joy of life are how I remember her.

With the increasing demands of John's job, our family life soon became almost non-existent. Finally realizing that was not how he wanted to live, he made a very difficult choice, one that most men are not willing to make. After thoughtful introspection, John recognized that Satan had him so consumed with the power and financial rewards of his job that he had minimized the value of his family. With a family photo in hand, he appealed to the upper echelon of his company, the top brass, to put his family first and he asked for a lesser position in the company. The result was the move back to Indianapolis after five years in Michigan.

We had been in Indianapolis for two weeks when Linda called to tell us about Alysa's illness. My first reaction was Lord, why move me here when I need to be a support for Linda? We don't always understand his timing...at first. I wanted to be there to support and encourage her. Instead, I had to support her from afar via our many phone conversations. When I would talk to her, I became consumed with the situation. At first I couldn't even understand what was going on. It was so hard to relate to what she was going through with her daughter.

Now, in retrospect, I realize why it was better for me to be removed. I would have been putting myself in the way. Perhaps Linda would have tried to lean on me instead of the Holy Spirit.

My job was to encourage her and pray for her. When she told me of the bizarre actions and the confusing things that where happening, it was God who put words in my mouth. In my own wisdom, I had no clue! But he always gave me something to say to Linda. I remember telling her to hold on to what God has done for her in the past. Hold on to his promises. He can get you through this, too.

When we received Linda's plea for us to drive to Michigan, we prayed in the car that we could be a comfort to Linda and Dave. We were not prepared for what we would see. We were horrified. Our memory was of a well Alysa and here she was with her eyelids fluttering over eyes that were rolled back in her head—not responding to anything. It appeared hopeless to us. She was a vegetable, we told our prayer groups in Indy. Alysa was on the weekly BSF prayer list and was being prayed for at our church as well.

Once, probably during the middle of Alysa's illness, God gave me an object lesson. Alysa had a very bad week. Her constant high fevers were not relieved. She was on my mind and in my prayers constantly. Adam, our son, was five at the time. He has a very high pain threshold, but that night he got very sick and experienced severe stomach pains. We were frantic, not knowing if we should take him to the emergency room or wait it out. Nor did we know how to comfort him. The pains subsided and he was fine. I believe God took me through that episode to re-unite me with what Linda was feeling. Since I was away from her, disconnected, I needed a renewed awakening of her physical pain.

It was shortly after that episode that Linda told me she was going to be obedient to Christ no matter what. When she told me that God told her Alysa was going to be well, I knew that the Lord was taking care of her. It may be hard for us, or others to understand entirely, because he did not speak to us. I know he gives us what we need when we need it…and that's what he did for her. He had given her peace. She walked so closely with the Lord, I said she was sticking to God like Krazy glue—she wasn't going to let go.

I think Linda daily empties herself and surrenders to God's will. Her commitment is solid. Often we have our own agenda for each day. Maybe we will think of what God has in store for us. Not Linda. She starts her day with God. She does not let an opportunity go by if she can share what God is doing in her life. Nurses, doctors, aides, janitors—they all encountered the unconditional love that Linda radiates. She made people look and see what God was doing for her daughter. She always had the love of Christ on her face. God used her in a mighty way.

CHAPTER SIXTEEN

Friends continued to aid the Conselyeas in their ordeal. Pastor Jim and Carol, Ray and Pat Thomas and the Conselyeas gathered in Grand Blanc at Damons for ribs on February 19th. After the much-enjoyed dinner they visited Alysa at Crooked Creek. With joined hands and spoken prayer around Alysa's bed, the parents felt the peace of having others care and pray for their daughter. Pat and Becky Toth, other "regulars," often made the drive to Grand Blanc. They shared stories of the antics of Christy, now away at college. Laneen, the engineer, frequently made the trek to Grand Blanc, too.

Linda, although embroiled in an ongoing trauma, recognized that life continued. She was never so selfish that she couldn't respond to others' joys and sorrows. She congratulated her sister, Carol, when she called to say she was engaged.

Tongue in cheek, she replied, "You mean you are going to marry him after dating for only ten years? Don't you think you're rushing it? Here. I'll put the phone up to Alysa's ear. You can tell her the good news."

Some might find Linda's attempts at normalizing her daughter's condition pathetic. But to Linda, holding the phone so Alysa could hear her aunt's voice was a chance to spark recognition or a reaction. Why miss an opportunity?

February 19, 1997
Day 283
9:30 p.m. Dad stuffing his face with pizza from Papa Romano's. Mom finally gets to go home. Alysa relaxing. H.R.=104. 24BPM. Going to feed Alysa and watch a movie. 9:45 Laneen in to see Alysa. Movie postponed. We've had a nice talk. 12:00 a.m. Laneen read Hebrews 3. 12:30 Laneen singing. Going to pray and go.

Since Linda partook in much of the daily care of Alysa, cleaning her trache site, her feeding tube site, and her soiled clothes and bedding, she was very much aware when something was wrong. It was with alarm that she called attention to the pass-port in Alysa's arm.

In a non-accusatory tone she said to the nurse, "I thought these pass-ports were supposed to be good for three years or more. This one looks like it is getting infected. It's all black and oozy. What do you think?"

"You're right. It doesn't look good. I think we need a doctor to take a look at it."

The port for medications did not last three months never mind three years. It had not received the proper care by the nursing staff who was unfamiliar with this particular surgical port. The doctor who had surgically implanted the port was livid.

In typical hindsight he told Linda, "I could have had the visiting nurse come to the nursing home to care for the port. I just didn't realize it wouldn't be cleaned properly. It is going to have to be surgically removed."

"The port is critical at this time because we just learned that Alysa finally gets to go to the Jerry Rush Hospital for her 24-hour evaluation/observation, and they need emergency access to administer drugs," Linda relayed, somewhat distressed.

"Don't you worry. We'll do a culture on the pass-port. Maybe we can keep it. If not, we'll bring her over to Mid Town and put a pick line in. I'll let you know right away."

"Thanks, Doctor. You've calmed me down a little."

Linda didn't stay calm for long. Alysa's Care Conference was scheduled for that very day. They reminded her that it was a fif-teen-minute meeting. Oh, oh she thought to herself. They know I've got major concerns. At her first opportunity she listed them.

"First, leaving the rectal probe plastic cover from the ther-mometer inside Alysa is inexcusable. It folded over and caused her undue discomfort. I would just like an apology from the nurse who did it instead of a denial. Second, Alysa had severe vomiting and I requested assistance and got none. Third, I have requested more stimulation for Alysa than the twice a week sessions. And last, the pass-port in Alysa's arm has become infected because it was improperly cared for."

Notes had been taken and heads nodded in affirmation, but not much was said...at the meeting. After Linda returned to Alysa's room, the nursing home director, who had not been present at the Care Conference, came to her.

Always pleasant, he approached Linda. "Mrs. Conselyea, I'm so sorry that you feel your requests have been ignored. I can assure you that our staff does the very best it can, but we all make mistakes. I would like to address your concerns."

"Please do," said Linda, sitting on the edge of the bed.

"The thermometer probe cover did no lasting damage. It was only a thin piece of sterile plastic...easy to lose. I'm sorry that happened. In the next week or so we are going to switch to using only ear-probe thermometers. About the pass-port site. I'm sure our nurses can handle that cleaning and maintaining procedure. It was just an oversight. And, we'll see that Alysa has someone com-ing in daily for large motor stimulation. Why didn't you let us know about these problems?"

"I haven't complained before because I didn't want Alysa to suffer any repercussions from my complaints. I didn't want her care to be jeopardized."

"I can assure you that would never happen. We have health care professionals that are proud of their work. There will still be a room for your daughter when you return from Jerry Rush."

He then informed her that the room referred to would be in a different wing of the facility. Since Alysa had no need of a venti-lator, and since the Conselyeas had been pushing to get the trache removed, she would not need to be on a higher care unit. The nursing home would be getting less money from her Medicaid, so they would provide less care. Money, again. The head of Respiratory had already asked who was paying for the ambulance ride to Jerry Rush. Linda didn't know.

From the valley to the mountaintop. Dave had his miracle in the early hours of the morning. He was preparing to leave Alysa to go home. He held her hand and talked loudly to her. She turned, looked right into his eyes and mumbled something. He asked her for a kiss and she leaned forward, puckered up, and planted a big kiss on dear old dad. His response? Praise the Lord!

Both Linda and Dave were inspired when a former Crooked Creek patient sought them out. He introduced himself as Jerry Crane. He was a big man in his late 40's.

"I was just visiting with some of the staff and they told me about your daughter. I thought I'd come and tell you my story. I, too, was in an apparent coma after a stroke. I had a trache and I had bouts with pneumonia. My brother was faithful in coming to see me every day. He would talk and read to me. I want to explain how I felt."

"Here, sit down," said Dave, dragging a chair away from the wall.

"It is very frightening to not be able to decipher between real conversation and talking on radio or TV. When I heard something on the news, I thought that was happening to me. And dreams seem like reality, too. I felt trapped because I couldn't express myself."

"So, that could be how Alysa feels, too?" Dave asked.

"Very likely so. I can only encourage you to keep talking to her, reading to her and stimulating her. You're doing all the right things. I wish you luck," Jerry said.

"Thanks. That's good to hear. We are trusting that our Lord is going to bring Alysa back to us 100 per cent. But we'll do all we can, too."

The pass-port could not be saved. The culture was positive and consequently hindered the chance of a new pass-port. A pick line had to be inserted instead.

Dave Conselyea paid for the ambulance trip to Jerry Rush Hospital. He accompanied Alysa on the surprisingly short ride from Grand Blanc to the east side of Detroit. This was the day they had been waiting for. The eagerly anticipated answers to

206

what was causing the seizures bombarded their minds and fueled their excitement.

Linda and Dave met the doctors while Alysa's stats were taken. The EEG technician got her all wired up right away. A strong, messy glue affixed the leads to her head. Dr. Barnett explained the procedure to the parents.

"Alysa will be monitored in every way possible: audio, video and the EEG. We will have EKG leads as well. She will have a team of specialists who can assess her by the various monitoring methods. You are actually part of the team. You can help us out and here's how. I'm giving you this strange-looking gray ball," he said, handing it to Dave.

"Whenever you see movement that you think is seizure movement, or even if you aren't sure, press the button on the ball and we all will come running to see what's happening."

The next day, March 11, the information sharing and discussion with the doctors continued. At first seeing Alysa "hooked up" and quite agitated concerned Linda.

Putting her at ease, Dr. Cameron told her, "We've reduced Alysa's seizure drugs, so you are seeing exaggerated movements today. Don't be overly concerned. We want to get a clearer picture of what is happening. Now, we need to know about her medications and her reactions to them. Also, could you please explain the exact movements she has made during her illness."

With the journals as backup, Dave and Linda easily listed Alysa's medication history. The explicit reactions were Linda's expertise. The eye, tongue, and mouth twitching and the arm movements were Dave's contribution.

The doctors' first assessment, based on their observations, surprised the Conselyeas.

"The movements that your daughter are making are not showing up as seizure movements," Dr. Barnett told them.

"Do you mean that the brain is not registering or is not causing the movements?" Dave asked.

"The EEG shows no disturbance, no unusual waves, during her moving episodes."

"So, what causes the movements?" Linda desperately wanted to know.

"My best guess is that the involuntary movements are from

the damage that the virus did to areas in the brain that control movement. EEG's don't always pick up deep seizures in the area of the brain that controls movement."

Stunned to learn of the registered absence of brain seizures, Linda mentioned, "Two other doctors, nearly 300 days ago, diagnosed herpes simplex. How can that virus cause all this?" Linda quietly demanded, waving her arm at Alysa, wired like an old-fashioned switchboard.

"We'll never know for sure. Once the herpes virus invades the brain, it attacks and manifests a myriad of symptoms. The drug Haldol can also cause permanent brain damage. We will just try to treat the symptoms we can identify."

Doctor Barnett discussed his treatment plan. "I want to use Klonipin and Lomictol, both anti-seizure medications. Then we will monitor her more closely to see their effect."

There was more to be monitored the next day. Alysa had pneumonia. New antibiotics began for treatment: Tobrymicin and Mezlocilin. While the respiratory techs worked on Alysa, Dr. Cameron spoke to Linda in the waiting room.

"We still are not seeing seizure activity. We want to take her off Phenobarbitol—cold turkey—in hopes that it may prompt a seizure or like affect, and thus help us pinpoint specific areas in the brain that may be causing her to have these myoclonic movements. Now let's go in and see your daughter."

He walked over to Alysa and held her hand and talked to her. He asked her how she was feeling and if she were comfortable. It pleased Linda to see the doctor treat Alysa as a human being and not just an object of medical interest. He seemed as if he had all the time in the world to spend on this case. What a gift, Linda thought.

Thursday, March 13
Day 305

8:30 a.m. Dad's been here all night. Dr. Cameron is in. He was able to see Alysa give me real kisses (ha, ha, Ken) and follow me with her eyes and shake her head yes in response to a question I asked. Then she started to cry after Dr. Cameron was explaining to me about her actions and what damage may have been done by the initial status epilepticus. Does she understand?

Dr. Simone, a fellow Neurological Specialist, found Linda that afternoon. "Good news," he said.

"Really, what?" Linda asked.

"I concur with Dr. Cameron and Dr. Barnett. Alysa's movements are not seizures. She's been off the Phenobarb for 24 hours without a seizure. When Phenobarb is stopped, the brain can react with seizure activity within the first five days. She may be off of it for good."

Alysa's pneumonia worsened and she was admitted to ICU, all the while being monitored by the continuous EEG. The doctors also had concern for a possible blood clot in her lungs. Feeling distraught, Linda recognized that at least Alysa was in the right place to receive the appropriate care.

On Friday, March 14, Alysa had an IV put in her left foot. A V-Q scan, radiation and air, detected no probable clot, so the Heparin was stopped. A Doppler study also verified no clot or obstruction. A nurse, Greg Piper, demonstrated chest percussion therapy for pneumonia.

As he rolled Alysa onto her side, he explained what he was doing. "First, I cup my hands like this," and he showed his hands as if he were going to gulp water from them. "Then I pound on her back with the blows coming mostly from the heels of my hands. This is very important to prevent pneumonia and to keep the mucus broken up. You need to see that this is done every two hours. Now I'd like for you to try it," he said to Linda, making room for her next to the bed. She tried it.

"Not bad. You are a little too timid. You can pound harder."

"Okay. I will next time. I promise."

He continued the therapy, beating on her back with rapid movements. Stimulated by the mild blows, Alysa became semi-alert. Her arousal was a beacon to Dave and Ken and they immediately moved to her side.

"Honey," Dave said. "It's Dad. Have you got a kiss for me?"

"Not so fast," Ken joked, "I'm the one who wants the first kiss."

Grinning at their competing for attention, Linda said, "You guys are goofy. Let Greg finish his session."

"That's okay. I just need to turn her on her other side for the next step." He turned her and discovered that an empty albuterol bottle (that had contained a respiratory medication) had been carelessly left in the bedclothes by one of the nurses and had worked its way between Alysa's legs. "I'll need you all to step out for awhile," he told them. The party was over. Later that night she was moved to the step-down unit.

On the evening of the 16th, Alysa's stats dropped very low. They bagged her, or gave her oxygen manually, and the stats went even lower. She was put on the ventilator again.

Ken was the attending loved one. "I really hate to see her back on that stupid machine," he told the nurse. "She's worked so hard to get off of it—twice."

"Don't you worry about it. This will just be for the night. She needs improved respiratory rates. She's breathing too fast at 50 BPM's. We'll go back to the oxygen cannula tomorrow," the nurse replied. "I also need to put in an art line. We can't get her blood gasses. Could you please step out momentarily?"

Confused by the term, Ken asked, "Just what is an art line?"

"An arterial line. It's like an IV, but it goes into an artery. It is a semi-permanent line."

Worried about Alysa becoming a human pincushion, he begrudgingly complied and stepped out of the room. When he reentered twenty minutes later, his stomach jolted. His poor baby had blood all over from the nurse's numerous attempts to do the art line. What else will you have to endure, he sadly wondered.

On St. Patrick's Day, Linda dressed in a green slacks outfit. Muttering to herself and talking to Alysa, she was fussing with Alysa's hair. "This glue is like cement. I don't know what in the world will get it out of your hair. These clumps are impossible to dissolve. I've used everything I can think of. Oh, does that hurt? I'm sorry, Honey. I'm doing the best that I can. Well, here, I'll leave this conditioner in for an hour and then try to wash it out."

The better she could make Alysa look, physically, the better Linda felt. She meticulously cared for her hair, nails, and personal hygiene. The tender care from mother to child equaled that of a new mother to her baby: unquestioning, unconditional love.

From the step-down unit, Alysa moved to a medical floor. Put right next to the Respiratory Department, she was in the ugliest room in the hospital.

No one could get well in this terrible room, Linda thought. And her roommate was a man! The doctor explained that the elderly man was blind and therefore Alysa's privacy was not compromised. But, Linda knew, the man had several young grandsons who visited regularly. Linda remained extremely uncomfortable with the situation. The medical nurses' unfamiliarity with a neurological case and the parade of grandsons caused her to increase her requests for a new room.

Tuesday, March 18
Day 310

6:50 p.m. Ken here. Dr. Cameron stopped by on his way home. He said the neuro floor is full, but as soon as they get an opening, they will transfer her. He wants to do an ENG to measure how long it takes signals to get from the brain to the muscles. This will help pinpoint where the movements originate in the brain. They also might do an MRI. He wrote a long note on her chart not to give Ativan for movements. He apologized that the non-neuro nurses would be dosing it. They were frightened by the movements. He also said that the pneumonia might be a result of Alysa's throwing up at Crooked Creek when Linda couldn't get help. Overall, he was very encouraging. Now, Alysa is kind of tense, eyes wide and to the right. Moving arms and mouth.

EMG and MRI cancelled on the 19th. The doctors wouldn't learn enough to warrant the tedious testing. Dave brought Chinese food for Ken, Linda and himself. Laneen visited Alysa at 10:00 p.m. Psalms, singing and praying lasted until past 11:30.

Dr. Cameron came in to discuss Alysa's case in detail. He told Linda his findings. He began with his opinion. "Actually, I think there are two different events going on. The initial virus is one event, and the second is hypoxia, or lack of oxygen getting to the brain. Alysa has been affected by both. I'm going to have the radiologist read Alysa's MRI from St. Vincent's and see if my suspicion is correct. I thought I saw something in the basal ganglia area. That is the part of the brain from where the myoclones can stem."

Ken was in charge again the next day, a Saturday. Linda and Dave had been kidnapped by their friends the Toths to go to

211

Frankenmuth for their world famous fried chicken dinners. He had a semi-confrontation with a new nurse. She was bagging Alysa.

"Mrs. Conselyea told me that Alysa is bagged before and after the suctioning, but not during," he ventured to state.

"That's not on the chart," she replied.

"But that's how it's been done before, I believe," he said.

"I'll call the doctor and see what he says," she responded.

After a few other disagreements took place, Ken learned that if you want something done, you'd better have the doctors write it down on the stupid chart! Alysa had so much suctioning recently that her trache site was raw and bleeding.

Dave's fortieth birthday coincided with the move to a neuro floor and a private room. It was March 24—Alysa's 15th day at Jerry Rush. Along with the four gifts stacked on Alysa's bed, the best present he received was the news that the discontinuing of Phenobarbitol was complete and no seizures had resulted from the cessation.

On March 25, Linda and Dave were conversing as they arrived. Dr. Cameron had told them that Alysa could be released to Crooked Creek.

"I knew this room was too good to be true. It's been her nicest room," Linda said.

Being supportive and encouraging, Dave said, "But aren't you glad that she's going back to the nursing home? We'll be closer to her. And it means she's so much better."

"Yeah, I know. I'm just not looking forward to training and teaching the nurses on the new wing at Crooked Creek."

"It will all work out, Babe. Don't worry about it"

CHAPTER SEVENTEEN

"Home again, Finnegan!" Dave said as they approached the reception desk at Crooked Creek Convalescent Home for Alysa's second admission.

Linda gave him a quizzical look, "Where did that expression come from and what on earth does it mean?"

"I don't know. My mom says it all the time. It just popped out."

A nurse, within earshot of their conversation, volunteered the answer. "I believe that one came from an old scout campfire songbook. It was a song titled "Michael Finnegan." Every line rhymed with Finnegan. Whiskers on his chinnigan, he drank ginnigan, he got thin again, and he would begin again. The song caught on and people created expressions that rhymed with Finnegan. 'Home again, Finnegan' was one of them."

"How did you know that?" Dave asked, incredulously.

"That's one of my hobbies. I have books and lists of old sayings."

"No kidding. Huh. You learn something everyday," Dave said.

Dave left for the office where he was now spending six to eight hours a day, unlike at the beginning of Alysa's illness when he spent zero. Linda, on the other hand, still had her life on hold. All normal activities of her life, with the exception of Bible Study Fellowship, had ceased to exist. Caring for Alysa was her

213

sole endeavor.

She met Alysa's new nurses and aides. Former nurses came in to say hi, and Tony from respiratory came in to reassure Linda. "In this wing, Alysa won't be checked on throughout the night, so I thought I'd set your mind at ease. I'll come down and see how she's doing."

"I'm so glad to hear that. I'll rest easier. Actually, I'm not feeling very well, myself. I'm going to head for home. Ken, Alysa's boyfriend will be here soon."

"Sure, I remember Ken. You take care of yourself."

Tuesday, March 25
Day 317

8:30 p.m. Nurse checked oxygen (first time all day). Low. Got Tony down here and he said she sounded chunky. He suctioned twice and got a lot of stuff out. Linda said Al coughing well all day. Maybe with the pneumonia she needs a little extra help bringing the secretions up before they collect in her lungs. I guess it's okay to suction when she needs it, but I hope they don't go overboard like at JR Hospital. But, of course, I don't want her to suffer any more damage from low oxygen. Too many things to worry about. No wonder Linda doesn't feel good! Glad Tony is checking on Alysa through the night. There is only one nurse for the entire hall. I do not like the sound of that. Also, meds have not arrived yet. Welcome to Crooked Creek.

The second team substituted for Linda the next few days. Linda Two, Ken, Nikki and Dave gave Alysa their full attention. It was hard for Linda not to see Alysa, but a bad attack of the flu made it impossible for her to get out of bed.

On Good Friday, March 28, Linda Two was with Alysa. She dialed Linda at home.

"Hi, kiddo. How are you feeling? Any better? Well, I thought you might want to tell Alysa hello. I'm holding the phone up to her now."

Alysa listened as her mother told her how much she missed her. She gave her phone kisses and said she'd see her as soon as she felt better. Alysa's new room had available plugs and space for Alysa to have her tape player set up and maybe a TV and VCR.

Dad would see to that.

An unfortunate incident happened that afternoon. An aide accidentally pulled the pick line out when she changed Alysa's wet gown. The nurse didn't seem to know how to put it back in so an LPN nurse was called in. Good thing. The site looked as if it were getting infected. Linda Two called Linda and told her what happened. They agreed that it was too bad, but hopefully Al wouldn't have to return to the hospital to get another surgical port.

On Saturday, Linda Two spent the day. Dave relieved her at 6:00 and Laneen arrived at 6:30 with some homemade pesto bread. Boy, did it smell good, Dave thought. They had the usual Laneen-led worship service with the reading of Luke, chapters 21-24, the Easter story, as the ever-touching end.

Easter Sunday is a joyous day for Christians. The resurrection of Jesus Christ is the historical fact and foundation of the Christian religion. Dave attended an early morning service so he could cater to his two girls. Linda was going to visit Alysa briefly, even though she wasn't entirely over her flu. Dave and Grandpa Rivers had tickets to the Red Wings hockey game that afternoon, and wild horses couldn't keep them away.

On April first, Alysa was dressed in her new Easter clothes, compliments of Grandpa Rivers, wrapped in blankets and whisked outside by Linda. Ken was now the sick one of the group and he wouldn't be coming in to see Alysa that day. Linda read to Alysa, gave her a manicure, and washed and blew-dry her hair. Just another day. Then Alysa threw up all over her new clothes. Linda washed her and got her into bed. Before leaving, Linda wrote a note to her daughter, "Alysa, may God protect you in a mighty way tonight. May you feel the special peace that passes all understanding. Love, Mom."

During the next month and a half the real Alysa emerged ever so slowly from her drugged and sickened cocoon. For the first time in a year, she waved at her mom when Linda entered her room. Alysa started to lie in bed in a natural position, no longer a stiff robot. She had a twinkle in her eye and had periods when she looked at people instead of staring through them. The tongue biting episodes were gone. And she experienced no brain seizures.

Setbacks, never welcomed, were tolerated. An unfortunate theft occurred. Alysa's high-top Nikes, worn to prevent unwanted foot drop, were stolen. Linda discovered the theft when she came in one morning to get Alysa dressed.

She remembered leaving them underneath the bedside table tray. "Where are your sneakers, Alysa? I know they were right here last night. I'll look in your closet."

She took everything out of the box on the floor of the closet and thoroughly searched the cubicle. "They're not here either. They are gone. I guess I'd better go tell one of the nurses."

Linda approached the nurses' station and told her tale. The head nurse reacted strongly. "I want you to file a police report. This isn't the first theft we have had. It shouldn't be ignored. I am appalled. How could anyone take her shoes? It makes me sick!"

Linda agreed and told the nurse how Alysa got those Nikes. "There is a friend of ours, Brent Gilbert, Uncle Brench to Alysa, who works a part time job once a month. He tithes that money to someone who needs it. His donation bought Alysa her shoes and some sweat clothes, too. So the person who stole the shoes actually stole God's shoes, not Alysa's."

That night at Alysa's bedside, Dave and Linda prayed for the thief. They forgave whoever took the shoes and hoped that he or she needed them more than Alysa did.

The peg tube, the name for the feeding tube, came out of her stomach and the balloon that holds it in place had burst. A trip to the hospital, by ambulance, for a new tube took only half a day. Physical therapy was put on hold. The excuse was that Alysa needed to show more progress. The real reason was lack of insurance.

As April neared May, the weather improved. Linda took Alysa outside for short periods each day. Alysa had high visual and audio sensitivity and needed to get reacquainted with the world outside her institutional facility. Linda would chat with her as they rolled along.

"Alysa, can you hear the birds singing? And hear that? Two boys just passed us on roller blades. I hear a dog barking. Do you? The driveway up ahead is getting a layer of asphalt. That doesn't smell so great, does it?"

Her one-way conversation was intended to provoke a response or recognition, but the stimulation proved overwhelming to Alysa.

When Pete Toth visited one day, he mentioned that one of the guys in his prayer group said he hoped that whoever stole Alysa's sneakers would get athlete's foot way up to his ankles. Alysa, hearing this, smiled a natural, funny smile. Alysa shook her head yes or no for her aides—and surprised the socks off them. She sat up straight one night when the phone rang and she hadn't done that for over a year. Her trache was still capped—the hole was covered where the respiratory hose attaches—and the ventilator and unnecessary equipment were removed from her room.

Then occurred the event for which Linda unmercifully chided herself. Linda: "I did the most stupid thing one night. There wasn't anyone to help me get Lysa to bed. I struggled, but I got her cleaned up and into bed by myself. One of the bed rails was down and Alysa fell out of bed and bumped her head. I felt unbelievably awful. I was worried about possible neuro damage. I called the nurse and a neuro check was administered. Alysa seemed fine. But I wasn't.

"I actually fired an aide. We were both working with Alysa, getting her cleaned up. This aide was mean, nasty and hateful. She was yelling at Alysa. If she was that bad in my presence, I could only imagine how she was in my absence. I made sure she never cared for Alysa again."

Sunday, April 27
Day 351
3:00 p.m. Mom here. Alysa decided to plant her feet firmly on the floor and wanted to stand. Nurse put her in bed instead. She slept while I worked on BSF. Ken arrived. We watched the movie "Phenomenon." Alysa woke up and gave Ken kisses! Lots of them. He said, "I love you" and in turn, Alysa said, "I love you," over and over. Ken was so excited. He called his mom. Linda Two called Nikki who called Carrie who called here for Alysa. Dave got two big kisses when he came in at 9:30.

The next day an aide walked into Alysa's room and as always, said Alysa's name.

"Alysa...."

Alysa responded, "What?"

The aide almost fainted!

The Conselyeas were given free reign of the Occupational

Therapy room. If it was not in use, they could have some privacy there. Sometimes they put blankets down on the floor for Alysa. Other times they took their VCR to watch videos. This time they were listening to a Red Wings game on the radio. Alysa was lying on a therapy table. Linda told Ken how Alysa had helped to wash her own face with a washcloth that afternoon. Dave went to his car to make some phone calls. When the respiratory therapist came in to get Alysa's pulse oxygen reading, Alysa woke up and said in a barely audible voice, "I've...I've got to go to...I've got to go to church!" Her first sentence—and Dave missed it. When told, he said, "Praise the Lord!"

On Tuesday, May 6, the trache was removed. It was a milestone day and an answer to prayer. The site was covered with gauze and tape—paper tape after a nurse was reminded about plastic tape. Linda took a picture of her daughter. Then they made rounds to show everyone that the trache was gone.

More good things happened the next day. Dr. Leech ordered a speech/swallow test, the breathing treatments were discontinued and Alysa insisted on standing. Ken was her supporter—literally.

While Ken was holding onto Alysa, Linda said, "Ken, which one of you is in better shape? You're sweating like a pig."

"Thanks a lot. You try it! This is hard work, but she doesn't want to stop."

After he was exhausted, Ken asked Alysa if she were ready to sit down. She nodded her assent. Realizing that this was a responsive time for her, Ken proceeded to ask her several questions.

"Do you want to go to Broad Street Café for coconut shrimp? Will you try to eat yogurt soon? Do your toes hurt?"

He got a head nod yes on the first two, and a shrug and half nod on the last. Ken and the family all looked forward to the time when Alysa could eat real food again. It would be a great sign of advancement. The real headway for Alysa was only a few days away.

*   *   *   *   *

Sunday, May 11, 1997, was the one-year anniversary of Alysa's first hospitalization. It was Mother's Day. Dave had borrowed Pete Toth's full-sized van to take Alysa where she requested to go—to church. Linda arrived early at Crooked Creek to get

Alysa dressed. An aide, Melanie, was so excited that although her night shift had ended, she stayed to help Linda.

She remarked on the clothes Linda had displayed on the bed. "Mrs. Conselyea, that sunflower dress is darling! Lysa will look so good in it. The straw hat and new shoes—they're perfect."

Alysa cooperated with her dressers and Ken and Dave situated her in her wheelchair. With their help, Alysa boarded the van and sat in the second row of seats with Ken next to her. They arrived at Faith Baptist Church at 8:30, partway through the early service.

Linda: "We couldn't exactly sneak in—four people with one in a wheelchair—are pretty conspicuous. We surprised Pastor Jim so much that he was speechless. He never regained his train of thought and finally gave up, left the pulpit and knelt down next to Alysa's wheelchair and prayed with her. Pete, Pat, and Becky Toth and Tom and Brenda Cox attended that early service so they could participate in the joy of that day."

Dave: "Although Alysa did not respond in a manner that would seem positive to an outsider unfamiliar with her situation, to her mom, Ken and me, it was an incredible day. She made a few sounds and sat through the remainder of the service without falling forward or slipping out of her wheelchair."

After church Dave led the charge. "Okay, we're off to see Mom and Dad. More surprises ahead."

They drove to the elder Conselyeas home and caught them as they prepared to leave to visit Alysa at Crooked Creek. They hugged their granddaughter with tears in their eyes. After a short visit, it was on to the Rivers house, Alysa's second home. Andy and Sylvia were still in church, so Alysa got situated on the couch to await their return.

"This is the best Mother's Day in the history of the world," Linda said. Her excitement ran rampant.

Exclamations bounced off the walls when the Rivers entered their home.

"Oh, Alysa, Alysa…I don't believe it. You're actually here," Sylvia blubbered.

Andy sat on the couch next to Alysa and took one of her hands in his. "Welcome home, kiddo. It's been a long time coming." Silent tears accompanied his greeting.

The clan rallied round. Linda's sister Vicki, her husband Matt, and nephew Sean, sister Carol and her husband Jim, Linda Two and Carrie all came over to share in the moment. Alysa was passing out "I love you's" to everyone. Her family lapped them up like thirst-starved puppies.

At 7:00 the time came to depart. Alysa was helped back into the van, but this time she realized where she was going. She began to cry and Grandpa Rivers helped to console her. It was 8:30 when the Conselyea trio returned to Crooked Creek.

"What a day!" Dave said.

"Wasn't it wonderful?" Linda said. "I can't stop praising the Lord for his goodness and faithfulness to us. Look how far he's brought Alysa. I know he'll continue to restore her health. Thank you, Lord, Jesus."

Ken got meaningful conversation and responses from Alysa on Day 370. Worried that Alysa might fall out of bed because she startled so when the phone rang, he missed the call. He called his mom to see if she had called. She hadn't but she was glad to talk to Alysa.

"Hi, Linda," Alysa said clearly and distinctly. "I love you." She listened some more and replied, "Okay."

Alysa hung up the phone, laughed and kissed Ken. He said, "I love you mostest."

Alysa shook her head, and said playfully, "No, you don't."

The "who loves who most" contest continued for the next few hours. Both won. Ken took her hand and for the first time she held it forcefully. It wasn't just a reflex. Finding it hard to leave while she was so lucid, he stayed till 4:30 a.m. He made the shorter trip to sleep at Alysa's parents since the next day was Saturday. When told of his success with Alysa, Linda masked her jealousy.

After the one-day outing, it was time to see how Alysa could manage an overnight at home. Linda had rearranged furniture and prepared the house for Alysa's homecoming. Alysa's mattress lay on the floor in the living room. Eagerness and trepidation vied to be uppermost of Linda's feelings. Alysa still was being fed through her feeding tube and received numerous medications. She was beginning to recognize when she was wet or soiled, but not in time to prevent it.

Ken and Dave brought Alysa home at noon on Saturday, May

17. Alysa made no particular response to being at home. She repeated words that others said to her and mimicked their facial expressions. Dave told her that Mom was making pork chops for dinner.

"Pork chops," Lys repeated. "Pork chops! PORK CHOPS!" she yelled.

Everyone laughed. The entire neighborhood now knew the Conselyeas' menu.

Dave had been watching the second game of the hockey play-offs. The Red Wings were playing the Avalanche. He came upstairs, announced the final score—Wings 4, Avalanche 2—and asked about the night's schedule. "Who's sleeping where?"

"I thought we'd take turns sleeping in the living room, either on the mattress with Lysa or on the sofa," Linda said. "Ken and Lysa have both been asleep for some time," she nodded to Alysa on the mattress and Ken on the floor next to her. "I messed up and gave her Lamictol when she was supposed to have Klonopin, so give her Klonopin at midnight. I'm going to bed."

"Okay. Don't worry about it."

Dave took a couch and dozed off and on. Alysa awakened at 4:00 a.m. apparently having nightmares. She seemed frightened and mumbled strange thoughts: "This place is a dump. I can't do anything. This is ridiculous." Dave wondered where she thought she was.

Alysa was the only one who got any sleep that night. Ken, Dave and Linda all slept with one eye open and one ear cocked. Sunday was spent caring for Alysa's bodily needs and physically moving her from one place to the other. She had moments of alertness and periods of rest and sleep. She returned to the nursing home at 8:00 p.m.

Linda: "I realized at this point that I was not physically ready to have Alysa at home by myself. Her needs were too great and I couldn't do it alone."

Many things were coming back to Alysa. She said to her mom, "I have two ferrets, don't I? Rocky and...I don't remember the name of the other one."

"It's Indy," Linda reminded her.

After Alysa's physical therapy had finally been approved, she started growing stronger from her daily sessions. Jane, her physical therapist, was sometimes calm and understanding and when necessary, goading and demanding. She and Alysa had bonded and had developed a deep relationship. Jane knew how to coax Alysa from her medicated dazes.

"Is your name Alicia?" she tauntingly asked Alysa.

Aroused from her stupor, Alysa stuttered quietly, "My, my...name is Alysa."

Jane knew how to deal with Alysa's periods of frustration and her mood swings. She told Linda some of the causes.

"Your daughter is still in a drugged state. Her inability to communicate is partly her illness and partly from the Phenobarbital. It can take more than a year to rid it from her system. Hallucinations and nightmares are also a residual result. Tell me, who is Billy?"

"Billy is her thirteen-year-old cousin. Why?"

"When she is really frustrated or riled about something, she starts yelling at Billy."

"What does she say?"

"Not much. 'Billy, no!' or 'Billy, you better not.' But she's angry when she says it."

"Poor Billy. He's really a good kid. Too bad she remembers him negatively."

"It's a phase. It will change. By the way, her strength is improving. She demanded that we keep her at the parallel bars forever the other day. We had three hours of P.T."

"You're doing a great job with her," Linda said. "We appreciate the kind of attention you are giving her."

"No problem."

Alysa had no problem expressing herself on May 28, when Linda Two and Nikki, Ken's sister-in-law, came to visit. Nikki later told Linda what Alysa said.

"If only I had gone to the doctor sooner," Alysa had told Nikki. "But I didn't have any money."

Linda felt very bad and thought if only she had known. Later that same day, Alysa told her mom, "I'm going to get a thousand dollars." That tidbit of accurate information sifted out of Alysa's memory.

"That's right, Lys. You were supposed to get that money at your court hearing last May. I forgot about it. I wonder what the status of the case is now," Linda said.

What Alysa remembered was a curious mishmash.

The next day, when Dave was with his daughter, Alysa was agitated. "I want to get out of here," she said. "Don't leave me."

"Lys, Honey. I'm here to stay," he reassured her.

Later that night she said, "I can't see."

Dave and Linda had been informed of Alysa's vision. The ophthalmologist had said that Alysa saw only in black and white. She had difficulty focusing and she had no left peripheral vision. She also had periods when she had no vision. This was one of those times.

"I'm right here with you, Sweetie. Your vision will get better in a little while. Why don't you just close your eyes and go to sleep."

Dr. Abraham came to see Alysa on June 2. He hadn't told Linda or Dave that he was coming. He left them a note: "I came by to see her. She looks great! First words I've ever heard from her were today! Dan Abraham." Then he was so excited, he called them to relate his feelings.

The Conselyeas were bringing Alysa home for part of every weekend. Once in one of her bad periods, she yelled, screamed, kicked, hit, and smacked anyone who came within an inch of her. Her family reminded themselves that it was the medication in control, not Alysa.

When she came home on June 8, she was more normal. Heidi, her pet dog, was also back and Alysa held her, smiled and kissed her furry face. The family bombarded her with all kinds of questions and she answered them all. Praise the Lord, Dave thought. She's almost back.

*   *   *   *   *

Interview with Steve Moffett

While driving the ten minutes from work at ITT (now Valeo) to his home nestled in an Auburn Hills woods, Steve Moffett sheds his manager's role to reveal that of minister by training, husband to wife Denise, care-taking dad to Stephanie and regular dad to younger daughter Samantha. The dirt lane's dense canopy of leaf-filled branches defies the afternoon's final rays of sunshine. But penetrating slivers momentarily glance off the hood of his car. Steve's life has known dark days, but he firmly grasps the

223

moments of sunshine.

Steve begins with his boyhood memories of his friend, Dave Conselyea:

Dave and I lived in the same Royal Oak neighborhood and attended the same grade school. One of my first recollections is of a street football game. We were probably second-graders then. We needed another player so we went to see if Dave would come out and play. We asked him and his reply was, "I can't. I'm watching the 'Music Man.'" We didn't know what the word incredulity meant, but it was written all over our faces.

We became buddies anyway and spent a lot of time at each other's houses. I'd spend the night at his house and often we'd sleep out in a tent. His mom was real nice and would fix us sandwiches and bring them out—like the commercial on TV. He in turn was always welcomed into our house. He was an unusually polite, perfect kid. When he spent the night at our house he asked my mom, "Mrs. Moffett, could I borrow your bathroom?"

I'd go with his family, year round, to Port Sanilac. We'd go mini-biking, fishing, snowmobiling and whatever seasonal pleasures were available for boys. He took me with him to Vacation Bible Schools. I was not a church-goer, but VBS with GI Joes was a novelty. When I was twelve, I accompanied Dave to a Jack Van Impe crusade in Bad Axe, Michigan. I was saved at that revival and I remember Dave's being glad for me.

During high school, we spent nearly every weekend together. When we were seniors at Kimball, Jim Vickey, Dave and I went to Florida at spring break. It wasn't exactly the typical beer and beach blanket scene. We stayed at my grandmother's. Dave, although quiet and conservative, liked the girls.

We attended Woodlawn Church of God together and helped with "visitation" on Monday nights. We'd go with adult "visitation" team members and call on visitors and new members to the church. Sometimes it was just the two of us fifteen-year-olds standing on some stranger's doorstep. Dave confidently steered the conversation while I inwardly supported him. We were also active in a youth group at the Ambassador Baptist Church.

We went different ways after high school. Dave went to Bob Jones University and I went to Midwestern Baptist College while I worked for Jack Van Impe in his personnel office. Even though

I didn't see Dave often, he was still my best friend.

I was dating Denise when Dave and I shared an apartment in Clawson, Michigan. We were definitely the odd couple. Dave was neat. I was messy. We shared a one-bedroom apartment. Dave always had his bed made before he left in the morning. I doubt if I ever did. Once we had dinner cooking in the oven and Dave left on an errand. He passed the fire trucks going in the opposite direction and said to himself, "Oh, oh, Steve forgot to take the casserole out of the oven." He was right. It was a temporary living arrangement because six months later Denise and I got married. Dave was our Best Man as I was his Best Man in his first marriage.

After his divorce, we seemed to drift apart. That was his wild oats period, which would be tame oatmeal for most. I was a fill-in, or substitute pastor at the First Alliance Church where I also led the youth group. Dave would come and sing for us. If you like Dean Martin's singing, you'd love Dave's.

When Dave married Linda, our friendship revitalized. We started playing golf together on a regular basis. Our jaunts helped my spirit because of the daily hardship at home. Stephanie, our oldest daughter, was born with multiple handicaps. She has cerebral palsy, is mildly retarded and is speech, hearing and vision impaired.

She no longer can walk, so she crawls or moves about via her wheelchair. Her only words are mommy, daddy and pizza. Dave has shown her love and tenderness all of her twenty-one years. He always hugs and kisses her and acknowledges her existence. My own extended family doesn't do that.

I was an acting pastor for ten years and I preached in more than 100 churches. I've asked God why Stephanie hasn't been healed, and my faith has been tested since her birth. Then I saw Alysa that first time in the hospital. My immediate prayer was, "God, if you won't heal Stephanie, please heal Alysa."

Alysa's situation looked pitiful. She was on the respirator, in a coma-like state and totally non-responsive. I visited almost every week and each time discovered that a new crisis had developed. I remember thinking will she die tonight or will she ever come out of it? My silent, unspoken advice to the Conselyeas was let her go—she won't get any better.

They told me now they knew how Denise and I feel. However, I thought their situation was much harder. My Stephanie had always been that way. Alysa had been a happy, vital Christian girl when she got sick. I found it much easier to accept Stephanie's condition than Alysa's.

I'm not an emotional person. I didn't cry when my parents died. When this happened to Alysa, I cried. Denise was deeply affected, too. After visiting Alysa, she would come home crying and literally, physically sick. She, too, felt that they were worse off than we.

Dave adopted a pretty even keel. "She's going to get better," he'd tell me. Linda's faith grew by leaps and bounds. She trusted God to heal Alysa and didn't give up hope. Her demeanor and actions were spiritually founded and I was wowed. I hosted a local Christian radio program and Dave was my announcer. We asked people to pray for Alysa. An untold number of listeners prayed for her healing.

I was heartbroken when she went to the nursing home. I thought that's where she'd spend the rest of her years. Linda was a stalwart of faith at that nursing home. She carried most of the burden during that time. Dave made daily trips, but he was trying to be at work, too. He worried about his aging parents, his business and money. He was always tired.

While visiting Alysa, I met Ken Komisarz. We prayed together on many occasions. His consistency and faithfulness toward Alysa overwhelmed me. I truly don't know if I would have had such loyalty to a girlfriend. I was so impressed with him that I hired him at ITT. We have established a kindred friendship.

Friends should help each other in times of need. I tried to just be there for them. I wanted them to know that someone cared. That's why I went to visit on Christmas Day. We had our family Christmas and were all settled in our household. I didn't want the Conselyeas to be alone. No longer that tongue-tied teenager, I'm good with people who are sick and hurting. My personal situation has honed my empathy for others.

Sickness exists on earth because of Adam's sin. God allows tragedy in our lives so we will trust in him. God allowed Job to lose everything—health, wealth and family—but Job refused to curse God. His faithfulness brought God's favor and his reward. I hold on to the promise that we'll understand it all when we get to heaven. The words from the hymn "When Morning Comes" give me peace and comfort. "We'll understand it by and by." I'm counting on that.

CHAPTER EIGHTEEN

Beach ball batting became the next big deal. Alysa had been given a big beach ball to toss around in her daily P.T. periods, an exercise designed to improve her coordination and test her following of commands. It was a big hit. Anyone who came to visit was asked to play catch. As Linda happily indulged her daughter, she wondered how many other things they would repeat as they had when Alysa was a child. Déjà vu.

Alysa had longer bouts of wakefulness. "Stand" was her favorite word and she wanted to practice standing all the time. Sometimes five people would assist Alysa at the parallel bars. During this healing period, Alysa's emotions were in turmoil. She became angry, combative and sometimes totally uncooperative. Nightmares and hallucinations also prevailed. The medications and the brain illness itself caused the outbursts, but that knowledge didn't make it any easier for the family or the staff to cope with them.

Her speaking was eerie and unassociated with anything one moment and then lucid and coherent at the next utterance. Although this unreliable speech was reminiscent of her early onset illness, to have her speak and respond at all remained encouraging.

Some of her unassociated comments were "Oh, I've been talking to my friends. You don't know them," "I want to get out the door," "I have to go somewhere for a few minutes," "I want to flush the toilet," "Why didn't you tell me?" "I wish I could get some sleep," "My friends are coming over and we can go to our rooms," and "She's a crybaby brat." The nurses and the aides enjoyed chatting with Alysa and would stop in her room between 10:30 and 11:30 p.m. for their nightly conversation. They loved seeing what more Alysa could do and say each day.

The nurses cracked up with laughter one day when they over-heard Alysa admonishing her father. Dave, alone with his daughter, enjoyed pushing her around in her wheelchair. He had just wheeled in front of the nurse's station and "parked" when Alysa surveyed her dad thoroughly.

In a very shocked voice, she asked, "Dad, is that a ponytail?"

"Lysa, Honey. I've been telling you that I'm not going to have my hair cut until you can do it. I've been waiting for over a year now."

"It's disgusting," she spat out, as if the word poisoned her mouth. "It might look good on some people, but it does not look good on you!"

"Gee, Honey. Too bad you can't tell me what you really think," Dave teased, adding, "nothing like a total dose of honesty along with your morning coffee, right?"

The nurses, thus given permission, laughed unguardedly.

Dave treated Linda to an early birthday dinner on June 12, at Mountain Jacks. He also wrote at the top of the journal page for Friday, June 13, 1997, "Happy Birthday To The Best Wife In The Whole Wide World." But on the actual day, Linda never heard from him. By 9:30 that night when she still hadn't seen hide nor hair of DLC, she was pretty upset. Three nurses walked down the hall each bearing three vending machine crumb cakes with light-ed candles. They sang Happy Birthday to Linda while she sat next to the sleeping Alysa on the floor mat. The couple passed each other at home—Linda going in to sleep and Dave, having been asleep, going out to be with Alysa. It wasn't the best of birthdays.

Dave and Linda continued to bring Alysa home for part of each weekend. It meant no sleep, lots of re-adjustment and hard work. But having their daughter home was worth all the effort. On Father's Day, June 15, Alysa visited both of her grandfathers. They welcomed her heartily.

On June 18, back at Crooked Creek, Linda and Dave were telling Alysa good night. As always, they had devotions and were ready to pray for Alysa. They were sitting on the floor mat and Alysa rolled over to their laps.

"Can we pray with you now?" Linda asked.

"Sure," Alysa replied.

"Do you want to pray with us?"

Without hesitation, Alysa began praying. "Dear Jesus, I love you, Lamb of God, hear my prayer." She paused. "Jesus, are you there? Do you hear me?"

In a firm, steady voice she sang the words, "Jesus loves me, this I know, for the Bible tells me so. Little ones to him belong. They are weak but he is strong, Yes, Jesus loves me. Yes, Jesus loves me. Yes, Jesus loves me. The Bible tells me so."

With tears coursing down her cheeks, Linda said softly, "Alysa. You remembered the words. You remembered those once forgotten words. Thank you, Lord."

The Conselyeas had renewed joy in their hearts that night. Alysa had prayed with understanding and evidenced her spiritual connection to God. From that moment on, she had repeated conversations with Jesus. "I love you Jesus. You're my friend." God had demonstrated his faithfulness to her and now she voiced it.

Dave tried to stimulate Alysa's memory every day. He'd hold up a bill and ask her what it was. "It's a fifty," she'd say.

"What two things do you remember most?" he asked one day.

"I remember all the times that we t.p.'d peoples' houses. That was so much fun! And remember when I got caught?" She would tell the nurses and aides of her escapades over and over. Her second fondest memory dealt with food.

"And, coconut shrimp. You must go to Broad Street Café and have their coconut shrimp. It is the best in the world. You've got to try it."

"Honey, you're making my mouth water down to my toes," an aide responded.

Friday's had Happy Hour. Linda decided they were going—regardless of the protest.

"Alysa, Honey. I thought we'd go to Happy Hour and hear the music...as bad as it is," she added under her breath. "I want you to experience some excitement and some noise. It's too calm and

230

quiet in this room."

No verbal protests arose, but Alysa still didn't like it. Her hearing had become hypersensitive, probably because she had been sightless for so long the nurses said, and getting re-acclimated to regular conversations and ambient noise irritated her.

Playing Bingo in the activity room wasn't so bad. Linda and Alysa each took a card and Linda would help cover Alysa's numbers.

"Oh, look Alysa. You just need N 34 and you'll win."

The second number called after that was N 34.

"You've won, you've won."

"Bingo," Alysa called out.

The prize was usually fruit. Red grapes this time.

"Umm. The grapes are good," Linda told her daughter. "I'm glad you won."

Bowling was another activity. Alysa stayed in her wheelchair using a special apparatus that allowed her to roll the ball. She did it! Of all the activities, movie days were her favorite.

On June 27, Linda overheard Alysa's end of the conversation as she talked to Ken on the phone. "Are you coming here today? You don't have to. So, are we doing something today? I'll do anything. I have to take a shower then. What? I don't want to watch TV. I'll talk to you in a little bit. I'll call you when I get ready. I love you. Okay. I'll let you go."

Linda took Alysa to the shower and afterwards got her dressed in her Pooh pajamas. And surprise, at 9:30 Ken did arrive. He told his Sweetie good-bye at 11:45. That same Sweetie was very combative the next time Ken spent any time with her. She was wet and didn't want clean briefs put on. Ken and an aide tried to get the dry briefs on Alysa. She yelled and cried and kicked. His patience nearly gone, Ken reminded himself that Alysa didn't understand what was going on.

Alysa came home for the July Fourth weekend. She sat in the yard overlooking the lake for a good part of the afternoon. Dave had planned an elaborate fireworks show but Alysa slept through the noise and the light show. Linda, however, was an appreciative audience so not all was lost.

Dave, Linda and Alysa had all been invited to a cookout at the Moffetts. They loaded Alysa into the Jeep and made an uneventful trip to their home. Alysa actually stood a lot, spoke to people and showed no agitation to be in an unfamiliar environment.

Thursday, July 10
Day 424

9:45 p.m. Ken here. When I arrived, Linda, Alysa and their builder friend John Bolan were waiting in the lobby for me. Lys was talking to everyone and she was standing up. Now she can brace the back of her knees against the chair and stand—no hands. Very impressive! She was wet so I took her back to the room. She pretended she was driving (she also pretended that we crashed). She was very cooperative when we changed her. I stood her up and Micky and Erin cleaned her up and put cream on her bottom. They said she was very red. Alysa did great. We just kept talking to her and explaining to her what we were doing and why. We remained calm and reassuring. She pulled up her pants by herself! Then she brushed her hair by herself. She also put her shirt on by herself after I got it over her head. She put her arm through and pulled it down. She settled down and after being fed, fell asleep. Carrie and Kelly had been with Alysa most of the day and they wore her out. After they witnessed all the things she can do, Micky and Erin wondered why Alysa isn't in Occupational Therapy.

Tonight on the TV hospital drama "ER," one segment showed a woman having seizures. First they gave her Ativan, then Dilantin, and then they put her in a Pentabarb coma because it was the only chance she had to survive. She had been seizing for half an hour. Her story ended tragically. Thank God for our miracle with Alysa!

The nurses would call Linda at home and report Alysa's accomplishments or problems. One such call was to relay that Alysa and an elderly resident, Eunice, were chatting next to the nursing station.

Alysa asked, "Do you have any children?"

"Yes, I have a daughter." Eunice continued to say how she never had any visitors.

The nurse was impressed with Alysa's caring expressions and the encouragement she was giving to Eunice.

"You know," Linda said, "Alysa used to visit Seniors in the nursing home and do that very thing."

The next day, as she ran errands, Linda answered a call on her car phone. It was Sally, one of the nurses. She chitchatted briefly and then delivered a bombshell.

"I'm afraid I have some bad news. Alysa was alone in her room in her wheelchair and we found her face down on the floor. I guess she tried to walk and took a fall. Nobody saw it happen. She is in an ambulance on her way to Women's Hospital south of Holly. She didn't respond to pain or pinching. She is non-responsive. She has a tiny slit beneath the eyelashes of her right eye. She must have stood and then clipped her head on the corner of the dresser," she concluded.

"Oh, no! Not another head injury," Linda said, the realization hitting her like a blow from a two by four. "I've got to call Dave."

*　　*　　*　　*　　*

Alysa was in the emergency room when Linda found her. Kneeling beside her, Linda prayed, "Dear Lord, protect this child and restore her to health. Please, God, show me that she is all right." A sick feeling of dread spread throughout Linda's body. Alysa opened and closed her eyes and remained totally non-responsive. A CAT scan was ordered and Alysa was taken to the machine. Meanwhile, Dave arrived to face this new ordeal with Linda. The two held hands and prayed fervently.

The nurse returned to the waiting room and approached the praying pair. "Well," she began. "I just had a lesson in pronunciation. I called your daughter Alicia. Without opening her eyes, she said to me in a very angry manner, 'My name is Alysa. A-L-Y-S-A. It's not that difficult.' Otherwise, she is still non-responsive. But she sure let me know how to say her name."

The Conselyeas' hope skyrocketed!

"Thank God! She spoke! I thought we might be back to Ground Zero," Linda said, elatedly. She couldn't help grinning at what prompted Alysa's speaking. That's my girl, she thought.

Next the doctor came in to tell them that everything looked good. No signs of brain contusion. He said they could probably go back to Crooked Creek shortly. Alysa was fitted with a neck brace and her arms were strapped down on the arms of her wheelchair.

233

The Conselyeas didn't like it and neither did Alysa. She awakened and with her hands in restraints, reached up and in microseconds, removed her neck brace. It remained off. Linda and Dave praised the Lord over and over for watching over Alysa. They did question why their daughter had been left alone in her room when she was supposed to be constantly monitored while in her wheelchair. In the car on the way to Crooked Creek, Alysa started talking.

Alysa was to be watched carefully for 24 hours. The next day she was ensconced next to the nurses' station so nurses could monitor her. Lysa engaged in one of her favorite games, Simon Says. As people passed her by, they would follow her directives and she theirs. "Simon says, touch your nose" a nurse would call out. Without any depth perception, Lysa missed by a mile, but she was willing to try. The director of Crooked Creek joined in the game, too. He knew that Alysa loved his Dodge Stealth and he had promised Alysa that when she walked out of there, he'd give her his car.

"Lysa, I've got some bad news for you," he told her.

"What?"

"I'm afraid I totaled my car yesterday. Now I can't give it to you. I'm sorry."

"Oh, that's okay. I don't want it. It was probably 20 years old," Alysa said, her old humor surfacing.

One night at the end of July, Dave picked up a pizza and brought it into the all-purpose room where Linda and Ken were teaching Alysa how to play cards. The pizza smelled wonderful.

"I'd like to have a bite of pizza," Lysa announced.

Linda and Dave looked at each other, and thought why not? He gave her a piece. She took one bite and started to gag. She immediately spat it out.

"That was disgusting! You tricked me. That's not pizza."

"Lys, Honey. It is pizza. I think your taste buds are fragile. You haven't had any food for fourteen months. Pizza isn't a good learning food. We'll try something bland next time," her mother promised.

Dave's prayer later that night would be for the Lord to give Alysa the capability and desire to eat and drink orally. The last few weeks of July had been particularly trying. Dave could see that Alysa's behavior was taking a toll on Linda. He had a plan.

After Lys was settled down and was sleeping, he called a family conference.

"I think we need to talk about what's bothering us and give each other a pep talk," he began. "Anyone want to go first?"

Ken volunteered. "I guess I'm a little put out by the false accusations. Alysa said I was sleeping with someone and I couldn't convince her otherwise."

"Oh, that explains what she yelled at me the other day. She thought I was you and was angry about my 'drunken binges' and my 'playboy lifestyle.' I was going to ask you about that," Dave said, grinning.

"See what I mean? And then when I'm trying to help her she indignantly says that she's not my responsibility. Then she accused me of sneaking a peek when I helped change her when she was wet. You can't win," Ken said. "The other day I had to show her my driver's license to prove who I was."

Dave nodded, understanding. "She doesn't always recognize us—you're right. She knows that Linda and David are her parents, but she doesn't always know that we are Linda and David. I hate it when she won't keep her clothes on. It's silly, because heaven knows modesty is lost in a place like this, but it is still conventional to wear clothing."

Linda had been very quiet during their steam-letting. She finally entered into the conversation.

"I know it isn't the real Alysa behaving so poorly. Her hallucinations drive her to do and say some pretty strange things. But I can't take the physical fighting. The kicking, hitting and biting—although seldom—sadden me. She's even had me in a headlock and squeezed my neck. It really hurt. She tells me to leave her alone all the time, too."

"Me, too," Ken said.

"And me," Dave said. "She asked me why I'm here all the time. I told her because I wanted to make sure she was getting good care. God has been so good to us and to Lys. She has come so far. This is a period that we will all laugh about in the future—if we survive. Why don't we just pray for strength and understanding and for God's continued comfort."

"And for thick skin," Linda added.

They bowed their heads and convened with their Lord.

235

Visitors came regularly. Pat and Becky Toth came on a sunny afternoon and after beach ball catch, they all did the Hokey Pokey with Alysa. She was dancing around and singing two of her favorite songs, "Everybody Loves Somebody" and "New York, New York." At each pause, she'd ask Pat and Becky who they were. Then she responded with "It's so nice to meet you." Everyone got a kick out of it.

Linda Two spent a day with Alysa and thought that her charge was going to sleep the day away. But Alysa awoke and became very active. Linda, the mom, was home making a cake and fighting white chocolate in the July heat. Linda Two was soon doing the Hokey Pokey and helping Alysa walk from P.T. to the dining room. Alysa talked incessantly. Back in her room, Alysa gave orders as Linda brought the wheelchair into the room.

"Okay. How are we going to do this?" Alysa asked. She answered her own question. She stood and held on to Linda and said. "Now just go sideways, easy, now down." She was in the chair. Linda was amazed at the advances Lysa had made.

On Friday, August 8, Linda informed her daughter of a conversation she had with a friend. "Lysa, you only met Kathy Evernham once so you probably don't remember her."

Lysa shook her head no.

"Well, I visited with her on Wednesday and she thinks that a book should be written about your illness and your recovery. What do you think?"

"I couldn't help. I can't remember anything about being sick."

"Alysa, I want to tell you what we have done. For over fourteen months we have kept journals that log everything that has happened to you."

Surprised, Alysa responded, "Really? You have?"

"Yes. And I think that maybe we could make a difference in other peoples' lives if they were to read this book. I don't think you know how hard it was on me to sit by and watch you hurt day after day. But then I believed that the Holy Spirit gave me a promise that you were going to be healed. The doctors at St. Vincent's Hospital said we should disconnect you from life support, but we thought that was not God's will for you. And look at you now. God has answered our prayers."

Alysa had listened intently to her mother's words. Tears had welled in her eyes and dripped, unwiped, on her shirt. "Mom, I didn't know. I'm sorry you suffered so much because of me." Alysa hugged her mom.

Linda whispered, "This hug and this moment make up for all the pain."

Alysa's five-year high school class reunion was the next day. Linda went shopping to see what she could find for Alysa to wear—if she went. That evening, an assessment was made and Ken, Dave and Linda got Alysa ready to go. The reunion was being held at Patrick's, a fancy restaurant in Auburn Hills. Once in the car, Alysa was concerned, for the first time, how her hair looked. She demanded to know her whereabouts, too.

"What road is this?"

"It's M-15."

"Now where are we?"

"We're on I-75."

She desperately wanted a bearing in her once-familiar world.

"Why am I wearing dress pants? Shouldn't I be wearing a skirt?"

"Lysa, you look beautiful. You look classy," Ken told her.

"How's my makeup?"

"Pretty as a picture."

The Jeep pulled into the parking lot, and Linda went inside to check things out. The former classmates were watching videos of their high school days, talking and laughing. Linda explained to a few people about Alysa's wariness in crowds. Brian Cooper offered to come to the car and bring Alysa in. He did, and the rest of the entourage trooped in. Alysa talked to some people and laughed at the videos. Before she could get agitated, the foursome retreated to the car. Friends came out to the parking lot, one by one, to visit with Alysa. It was a great occasion.

Ken visited his Sweetie Saturday afternoon, August 16.

Knowing they wouldn't go, he asked anyway. "Say, do you want to go to the Dream Cruise?" It was Motor City's fixation with old cars parading down Woodward Avenue in royal splendor.

"Sure, it sounds good to me."

"Well, maybe instead I'll just tell you how I feel about you." He shared some mushy tidbits and sweet-talked to her.

Starting to cry, Alysa said, "No one has ever said such wonderful things to me before." Her feet were bothering her so she removed her shoes. Then suddenly, she made an announcement.

"I've got to go potty. Now."

With the wheelchair facing the wrong way and the bathroom door blocked, Ken tried to get the wheelchair over the mat.

"No, I want to walk to the bathroom."

A few rumba-like maneuvers were attempted with no luck.

"Come on, Sweetie. Get in the chair and let me take you."

"I have to go right now."

"Okay. Okay. Here, the chair is ready.'

She sat. He pushed. Ken helped her lower her panties, assisted her on the toilet, and she went! It was a first.

"I want a shower, too," Alysa said as she started to strip off her clothing. "Start the water."

"Whoa, girl. That's outside of my comfort zone."

It took all of Ken's persuasion powers to kill the shower idea. Finally Alysa discarded the notion and allowed Ken to take her back into her room.

Alysa slept for awhile and when she awoke, she thought she was an actress in a play. She attempted to seduce Ken who, in her mind, was Hitler. She had to convince him that he loved the Jews. He didn't mind the seduction part, but he preferred reality.

"Okay. That was weird. Now, you be Alysa and I'll be Ken, all right?"

They laughed over the episode and decided to tell her parents when they arrived. They talked about many subjects, and Alysa noticed that Ken was writing in the journal.

"I want to write," she said.

"Fine. Let me help you."

"Should I write in cursive or print?"

"Let's print."

Ken helped guide Alysa's unsteady hand on the page while they printed her name.

"I want to try it by myself."

With hard concentration, Alysa painstakingly wrote those letters for all the world to see—the name that was so special to her: A-L-Y-S-A.

Alysa became more observant of her surroundings. "Mom, you've let your hair grow long," she said as they were driving in the car. And at her evaluation at the state social worker's office she chatted up a storm and confided to the woman, "You know, my dad is really very conservative. The ponytail look isn't him at all." They discussed her bad dreams and the social worker explained to Alysa that although they were dreams, they would seem very real to her. Alysa received some consolation from her words.

Linda had personally been decreasing the Klonipin dosages, but the official order to do so started on August 17. The resultant effect on Alysa was dramatic. Besides being alert for longer periods, the incessant itching lessened. Alysa spent that day at Grandma and Grandpa Rivers. The elder and the younger Conselyeas drove two hours north to Aunt Martha's 90th birthday celebration. Both sets of grandparents and Linda and Dave spent time with Alysa after the trip. All were thrilled that Alysa continued to recognize her need to urinate and could make it to even an unfamiliar bathroom. Before they left, Alysa asked for everyone to pray for her. "The evil spirits don't bother me at home—just at Crooked Creek," she said.

The next day, back at that scary Crooked Creek, Alysa asked Linda, "When will Dad be here? I've had enough of this place, and I want to go home. Let's call Dad. I want him here."

"Okay, let's call him," Linda said.

Dave left his office in an instant and headed to Crooked Creek. On the way, he stopped and got a vanilla milk shake for Alysa. He arrived, and handed over his surprise.

"It doesn't taste like vanilla," Alysa said after sampling a few sips. "Why does it have that cover on the top and a straw in the middle?"

She didn't go home that day, but was consoled to have her dad there with her. She wouldn't let him feed her the Jevity in her feeding tube.

"I want something real to eat. Take me to the doctor for food," she said.

Alysa's interest in food was growing. They went to watch bowling and Alysa smelled the popcorn.

"I'd like to try some," she mentioned.

Linda gave her three kernels that Alysa carefully chewed and swallowed.

"Now I'd like some orange juice," she announced.

Linda went across the street and bought a bottle of orange juice. Alysa poured it into a cup and drank it. The whim of a child isn't always met with such instant gratification, but for Alysa to have a need that could be so easily met thrilled the parents.

Back in her room after washing her hands in the sink, Alysa said, "Could you go and get me some chicken? Any kind. I'm not picky."

"Soon, Honey, soon."

To divert her attention from forbidden food, they played cards. Ken helped Alysa with Blackjack, but she shushed him when she thought he was revealing her cards.

"How much money do you have?" she asked her mom.

"A dollar."

"Well, you're going to have to go get a job to pay me back," she boasted.

'That good, huh? We'll see."

That night as they had devotions and Linda began to read Psalm 91.

"Wait, stop. Why would God protect me and care about me when there are thousands of people in this world?"

"Lys, he loves all the world and especially those who love him."

"I want to say the Lord's prayer. I want to hold it in my hands."

"How about if you hold your Bible. The Lord's prayer is there—in Matthew 6."

They said the prayer together and soon Alysa fell asleep holding the Bible in her hands.

The phone became a constant companion for Alysa. Easily encouraged to call people, she called Miss Brenda, a very surprised Brenda Cox, and wished her a happy birthday. The next call went to Laurie Hall, and on a roll, she phoned Linda Two, and Grandma. With her birthday coming up, she called former high school friends and friends from Bardha Salon.

Two of her good friends called her and asked if they could visit the next day. Lysa informed them that she'd be at home on Saturday—could they come there? Jennifer Forston and Noel Winters brought photo albums to share with their friend. The three of them sat with their heads bent pointing and laughing at the pictures. Their kind gesture eased Alysa back into her world of faces and places. Girl time and girl talk were therapeutic for Alysa and heartwarming for the observing Linda.

"Smashing" describes Alysa's twenty-third birthday party. The staff and residents at Crooked Creek celebrated along with an outpouring of guests. With her dad at her side, Alysa was escorted into the dining room where she was greeted with applause and beaming smiles. Cindy and John Schmidler and their son Adam missed a family reunion to be at Lysa's party. Cake, food, gifts and Kareoke singing filled the halls. Lysa spoke to and thanked every person who came.

Dave penned a familiar comment in the journal that night. PRAISE GOD!

CHAPTER NINETEEN

Dave brought Alysa home on Wednesday before he left for his annual golf outing at Boyne Mountain on Thursday, September 4. Alysa slept in her parents' bed and he was the overseer. In the night Alysa had sprung a leak, so to speak, and Dave changed her and all the bedding.

As he headed for the washing machine, he thought, "I'm so grateful to God for her healing. I could care less if she wet the bed from here to eternity."

Ken planned to help Linda with Alysa over the weekend, but needing moral support if not physical and emotional support, she took Lysa to Grandma Rivers on Thursday instead. Although her eyes still wouldn't focus for her, Alysa watched her favorite movie, "Annie," over and over. In conversation with her grandparents and her mom, Alysa pursued some heavy subjects.

"What is my purpose in life?"

"Your purpose is the same as everyone's. To honor God and live as the Bible teaches," Sylvia told her. "He wants us to do his will."

"But I'm only one girl. What good could I do?"

"Lysa, Honey," Grandpa said, "your life has already touched many people. So have your parents' lives. You have no idea how many people watched how Linda and Dave reacted throughout your illness. And then your recovery...." Grandpa got choked up at this point. "Your recovery is a miracle," he finished.

Dave called home on Saturday to check on his girls.

"How's it going?" he asked.

"Pretty good. It is so wonderful having her home. Dave, I don't want to take her back to the nursing home."

"Then don't. You've got Ken there to help, don't you? Why don't you get her meds and Jevity from the Creek and keep her there."

"I think I will."

Meanwhile Dave had a crisis of his own. He knew that his smoking habit had bothered his wife and daughter for years. He knew, too, that smoking hurt his testimony as a Christian. When Alysa entered Crooked Creek nearly six months ago he told God that if he let Alysa walk out of that place, he'd quit smoking. Dave thanked God for Alysa's amazing progress. Now it was pay up time.

Dave's non-Christian golf buddies were drinking wine when he returned from the phone call. Dave savored one last cigarette.

Paul taunted, "Hey, what are you doing smoking? I thought you were going to quit this year. Aw, you couldn't quit if you tried."

"Yes, I can. I promised God I would quit."

"Tell you what. If you quit this second, I'll pay for next year's golf outing." He thought he had made a pretty safe wager.

Handing over his cigarettes and lighter, Dave accepted the offer. "Here. You've got yourself a deal."

Later, Dave acknowledged that he hadn't been fair to Paul. The Lord took away his desire to smoke, Dave said. He hasn't smoked since that very moment.

Linda, Alysa and Ken attended church that next morning. At the end of the service, Alysa went forward to kneel at the altar. Pastor Jim hurried to her side and prayed with her. He stood and gave a brief synopsis of her story and asked who would commit to pray for her that week. When nearly every hand in the audience of over one thousand was raised, Alysa cried her heart out. Linda did, too. People came to speak kind words and quiet prayers to Alysa.

Tears dried, they went to L.A. Café for breakfast. Heidi came to the car and personally escorted Alysa into the restaurant where she once worked. Still getting her food from the feeding tube, Alysa wanted to at least try some blueberry pancakes. Later that day, at Ken's brother's birthday party, she tried an olive, piroges and corn on the cob!

"Boy, only God could make something taste this good," she said as she chomped on the ear of corn.

Monday morning Linda received a phone call at home that Alysa was not yet discharged and she needed to return to the nursing facility. The doctor said that after a 24-hour documented observation, she could be released. The nurses needed to record the results from the reduced medications and fill out reports and other mandatory paperwork. So Lysa and her mom trooped back to Crooked Creek. The official day of dismissal would be Wednesday, September 10, 1997.

Lysa engaged in her normal routine of whirlpool bath, P.T. and O.T, but with a heightened response from the personnel. Everyone had words of encouragement and best wishes for her health. Jane, the physical therapist with whom Alysa had so firmly bonded, found parting very difficult. They prolonged their workout with pats, hugs and a few tears. A new pad for her going-home wheelchair was presented with much ceremony.

Dave spent the night with Alysa on Tuesday the 9th.

"What's this?" he asked the next morning as an aide approached with a fully loaded breakfast tray.

"Wouldn't you know it? Breakfast in bed. In the 170 days we've been here, this is the first time I've seen anything like this. Thank you so much!" He dived into the French toast, scrambled eggs, cereal, orange juice and coffee while Alysa continued her sleep on the floor mat.

"You're very welcome. We are going to miss you folks," the aide said

"We will miss all of you, too."

Wednesday, September 10, 1997
Day 486

8:00 a.m. Dad here. After being here for so long, since December of 1996, I feel mixed emotions about leaving this place. I have joy over finally getting our girl home and away from all of the noise and confusion, but I also have sorrow over leaving so

244

many caring and good staff. It has been a lengthy and exhaustive experience, but through it all we can see the hand of God at work. Who would have known the journey that God had in store for us since May 12, 1996. I give him thanksgiving as we journey into the future with him guiding our steps. Praise be to God.

Instructions were given to Linda about Alysa's drugs and the feeding tube. The dietitian advised that it remain in place until Alysa was consuming 1200 calories of regular food. Boxes of personal belongings were hauled to the cars. The discharge papers were signed.

At 2:00, a showered, dressed and smiling Alysa walked into the dining room to say good-bye. Jane stood by her side and Dave took pictures of the farewell group. Residents and staff, reluctant to let her go, touched her hands and patted her arms. Cheerful and subdued at the same time, they bid her farewell and told her to have a good life. The Conselyeas exited to cheers and waves and climbed into their two fully-loaded cars.

Dave and Alysa rode together and Linda drove separately. Per Alysa's request, Dave stopped at McDonalds and picked up dinner—a fish filet, fries and a Sprite for Alysa to taste. They took their edible treasure home and gathered around the kitchen table.

"Lys, Mom and I have prayed for sixteen months that one day we would all share supper around this kitchen table and eat together as a family. God answered those prayers."

Beaming, Linda added, "Lysa, I just can't believe you are finally home."

"Home," said Alysa. "I think that is the best word in the entire English language."

*   *   *   *   *

Interview with Alysa Marie Conselyea

A personable, cheerful, competent young woman crosses the threshold into the entryway. The date is October 14, 1998. Only the slight hesitation step of her right leg suggests any hindrance. Her social graces intact she compliments the décor and is then ready, eager even, to tell her story. "After all," she had said to a friend on the phone the night before, "The book is about me." Just one year earlier Alysa had come home in a wheelchair with mul-

245

tiple limitations. No one could have predicted then that she would be capable of verbally contributing to her story.

Alysa, in her own words:

After high school I attended Bob Jones University merely because a lot of my friends were going. I didn't really like it because it was too strict. I wasn't rebellious like some, but I did get some demerits—for being late to class. I followed the dress code and the other rules, but mainly just went along with the flow. I felt like I was not following my goals in speech and communication, so I left after my freshman year.

Back at home I became engulfed at my mom's candy shop in Clarkston. She needed help and couldn't pay a real employee, so I became her shop person. I put in long hours from nine in the morning until late at night. I was cashier and worked the coffee and cappuccino machine. I liked the interaction with the customers. I am a people person, so that was fun for me. After the shop burned, we were all distraught.

Next I tried a semester at Oakland Community College. I took the pre-requisite courses, but I didn't continue on at that time.

I then got a job as a waitress at L.A. Café in Waterford. That position opened my eyes on the world. I had been used to being around Christians, in high school and at college, and now I was introduced to people from all different walks of life. The clientele at the nighttime coffee bar comprised young and old, normal and strange, and some outright bizarre folks. In fact one of the waitresses was a professed witch and Halloween was a real holiday to her. She also claimed to be a homosexual. I was thrown off by her beliefs, but I held to my own beliefs and values. The owners, Heidi and Darren, treated me as a peer and we even socialized together.

Realizing that I was bouncing around and not meeting goals I had set, I determined to pursue something that had always interested me. While I was at Bob Jones, I repeatedly had requests to do my roommate's hair. I had a flair for "up-do's" and fancy styles and loved doing it. A couple girls there were planning to leave school and go into cosmetology school. That planted a seed and the idea germinated.

Grandpa Ralph knows everybody and every business in the Royal Oak area and he suggested I enroll at David Presley's

Beauty School. My other grandparents chimed in and said I could live with them to make it easier to go to school. So it was all set. The very first day I went, I liked it. There were about 29 girls in my beginning class. The course requires 1,500 hours of training in hair, nails and facials.

To get acquainted and improve speaking skills we were all to give a demonstration speech on any topic. I chose how to be a sorority girl in the style of a Saturday Night Live skit. I did the walk and the talk, and putting on airs, I introduced myself as a "Kohpa, Kohpa, Kohpa." I got an A. Many of us became friends and we had a great time.

We worked on manikins at first. Then we worked on clients who liked getting their hair done for a small fee. We'd fix the woman's hair and an instructor would check our work. After 1,000 hours of training, we would advance to the main salon where we would work with observation but without on-the-spot critique.

Nikki Komisarz and I became good friends. She told me about her brother-in-law, but I had little interest. I had lots of friends from L.A. Café and I wasn't really interested in dating. Her husband, Matt, had a party and I was invited. I met Ken, we talked and he later asked me out. He was pretty easy-going and very nice so I said yes when he asked me for a second date. After that came a third and a fourth and the rest is history.

Graduation from beauty school was low-key—no function—no cap and gown. One of the girls said she was going to bring in some stuffed grape leaves and a party mushroomed from there. Mom made one of her chocolate tortes. So we created a festive last day. All of us were moving on to salons for employment.

The Bardha Salon in Birmingham had been my mother's hair salon for many years. She inquired about openings and I followed up and was hired as an assistant to Bessa. An assistant sweeps up cut hair, organizes the appointment calendar, fills shampoo bottles and other slave jobs—for very little money. I watched and learned as I did my work. Debbie, another stylist, spent her weekends as a Redken representative going to hair shows, giving demonstrations and teaching classes. The extra money appealed to me and I mentioned that I was interested. She arranged for me to go along to East Lansing to her next hair show. I went. She introduced me to the director and I told him how great I thought the Redken product was. After that trip, my memory is pretty blurry.

I remember having a seizure in Ken's car. I remember he pulled over. The next thing I remember is coming home from being sick. I didn't realize that sixteen months had gone by. Actually, the first people I remember being with were Jennifer and Noel, who visited me at my house.

Physical therapy and occupational therapy, necessary parts of my recovery, became overwhelming to me. I rebelled. I didn't want to go. Now I've changed my mind and I'm having P.T. and O.T. and S.T. (speech therapy) on a regular basis. If I'm to get my right leg working normally, I have to keep it up. I do stretches, stairs, the treadmill, balancing and more. I've started walking on our road to increase my confidence and to exercise my leg. I'm supposed to wear my ankle brace every day, too. Working with Hema, my therapist, is ideal; I'm not self-motivated.

My current goal is to get my beauty license renewed and get back into the hair field. In the meantime, I'm cutting my friend's and my parents' hair, practicing driving with my dad and relearning skills in O.T. and S.T. We do memory games, math questions, cook and bake and a lot of computer work. The occupational therapist didn't like it when I didn't check off each item on the recipe when I made cookies or brownies. I didn't need to. It was easy.

For awhile I just sat at home and played solitaire or other games. I was attracted to all the food I hadn't eaten for so long. Everything tasted so wonderful. Too wonderful. When I left the nursing home, I was a size six. That's too small for me, but I've put on too much weight. I went to the doctor recently and stepped on his scales. I cried when I saw the number. I'm not this size either. I'm somewhere in between. The walking, aerobics class and the P.T. will help while I decrease my calorie intake.

I would not have gotten through these months without the help of God. I know prayer played an enormous part in my recovery. I remained on the Faith Baptist Church prayer list that entire time— all 16 months from when I first got sick to September 10, 1997, when I was released from the nursing home. Now people I've never met come up to me and tell me that they prayed for me. I thank them profoundly for their prayers.

I'm thankful, too, for the prayers of my parents, my family

and people I'll never know. Graduates from my high school all had a life verse from the Bible that they claimed. I never really had one. But now I have a picture above my bed that shows an angel. Muscular and strong he holds the hand of a sleeping child. The words written at the bottom of the picture are paraphrased from Psalm 91, verses five and eleven. "You no longer need to be afraid of the dark anymore, nor the dangers of the day...For the Lord has sent a Guardian Angel to protect you, and to go wherever you may go."

I have always been a believer. I was saved when I was only nine-years-old and in a fifth grade Sunday School class. I knew Jesus and that he was real. God has always been there for me. I wonder why I got sick, but I haven't blamed God or gotten mad at him. As for those lost sixteen months? Thank God, I don't remember them. But even better, I never lost my faith. Isn't that a miracle?

EPILOGUE

Tuesday, October 28, 1997
Day 535

Today was a celebration day. I, Linda, took Alysa to MIND, Michigan Institute of Neurological Disorders. Dr. Corbin, Dr. Owens, and Dr. Abraham all were there. They wanted to see how Alysa was doing. I wasn't sure how she would react. I told her that these people were her advocates, her supporters and friends. I asked Dr. Corbin if she remembered my telling her in the parking lot so many months ago that God would heal Alysa. Her reaction, "Yeah, right." Dr. Abraham greeted us with his usual warmth. Dr. Owens, throughout our visit kept saying, "This is truly a miracle." All were trying to speak to Alysa at once. She answered their questions, and even kidded around with them. The only question she couldn't answer was "Do you remember what happened that weekend in East Lansing?" To them that was crucial. It's their need to understand. I believe she may have had her first seizure in that bed while her roommate was sleeping. I'm past that now. Instead, I just praise God daily for Alysa's life and for the joy of having my daughter restored.

Interview with Linda Conselyea

Today, a year after Alysa's homecoming I believe the doctors needed to see what God could do. Alysa was brought into their

250

lives for that reason. During that visit a year ago, they all registered unreserved joy and compassion. Dr. Abraham hugged Alysa
and told me that everyone in the hospital continued to pray for her.
Isn't that wonderful? An entire hospital believes that God answers
their prayers

As a Christian parent I better understand how God, our heavenly Father, must have felt as he watched his precious, innocent
Son, Jesus Christ, suffer in agony and pain on the crucifixion
cross. He couldn't eliminate the torture because his master plan
for the world's salvation resided in that pain. Christ suffered
because of our sins.

Daily, I watched Alysa suffer as she was poked, prodded and
trapped in a body that couldn't cry out for relief. As her mother I
couldn't shield her from or remove her pain. Alysa's illness was
God's master plan for her. I knew that Alysa personified his perfect will and his eternal purpose.

Once I completely trusted him for Alysa's life, I encountered
the peace of obedience. The opinions of other people had no cre-
dence. I relied solely on God. Today I remain grateful to God for
allowing us to experience phenomenal blessings during even the
darkest days of Alysa's illness. I give Our Lord God all of the
praise, honor and glory for the physical healing of Alysa and especially for the many lives that she touched.

Verses five and six in Proverbs 3 say it best. "Trust in the
LORD with all your heart and lean not on your own understanding; in all your ways acknowledge him, and he will make your
paths straight."

Mere mortals can never fathom the plans of God. But if we
give him praise in all ways—even for the bad times—he will
direct the way. And he did.

I have no worries about Alysa's future. God has already used
her in a mighty way. Whatever he chooses for her is her destiny. I
am content knowing that "God is at work in her, both to will and
to work for his good pleasure."

Interview with Dave Conselyea

Today is Day 822, or 2 ½ years, since Alysa first went into the
hospital because she felt "out-of-it." If anyone had told me on
May 12, 1996, that Linda and I were going to spend the next 16

251

months in a combination of six hospitals and two nursing homes with our daughter near death, I would not have believed him. Nor would I have believed that anything good would have resulted from this terrible experience.

Her illness, her miraculous recovery, her daily improvements—mentally, physically and spiritually—proclaim that God is able. If I could have controlled her destiny, I never would have let her suffer and would have shielded her from her agony. I begged God to let me suffer in her place. One of my prayers throughout Alysa's entire illness was that she would not remember all of the bad things that happened to her. She was in such pain, discomfort and misery so many times. It broke my heart to see her suffer so much. I prayed, "Please God, erase that pain from her memory forever. Just as you erased our sins with the death of your Son, keep her pain as far away as the East is from the West."

He is a faithful God. He honored and answered that prayer. Today Alysa has zero recollection of anything that caused her pain. She only knows some of the good things—the great medical people, the faithful prayer warriors—because we have told her about them.

Only by hindsight can I see God's incredible plan to bring so many people together to pray for and be touched by Alysa. But I believed then as I do now what the apostle Paul says in Romans, "And we know that in all things God works for the good of those who love him, who have been called according to his purpose."

Alysa's trials caused her boyfriend to accept Jesus Christ as his Savior. Only God knows how many other people were saved through this ordeal. I pray that even more will come to know God through his Son, Jesus Christ, as they learn of our remarkable journey.

My simple prayer for Alysa's future is that God will continue to live through her life. I thank God daily for sparing our daughter and for renewing my heart to my priority—my family. Praise the Lord!

Interview with Ralph Conselyea

I had Catholic friends and Jewish friends who were praying for Alysa along with us. That's all any of us could do. Just pray.

And look what happened. She's getting better every day. It's a miracle.

Interview with Pastor Jim Combs
Some folks have asked why something like this happened to Alysa, a good Christian girl. In Genesis, the Lord looked upon Abel and his sacrificial offering with favor. His brother, Cain, in jealous anger killed Abel. Why did Abel die at the hands of his brother? He had honored God, not offended him. The Hebrew word for Abel is vapor. God says in His word "life is like a vapor." He wasn't surprised by Abel's early death nor did he prevent it. Abel is remembered throughout the Bible as one who knew what God expected. In Hebrews it says, "By faith he was commended as a righteous man, when God spoke well of his offerings. And by faith he still speaks, even though he is dead." Abel was the first martyr for truth.

Throughout the history of mankind, godly men and women have had bad things happen to them. Job in the Old Testament was such a person. God complimented him and called Job perfect and upright in the Word. Then Job's life turned to ruin. With his health tested, his finances wiped out, and his family extinguished Job questioned why God let this happen to him. When he finally understood that knowing God far outweighed knowing answers, his riches, his health and a family to love were restored.

Suffering can shape us for service to others, can be a result of bad decisions, can be an attack from Satan or can just happen. Alysa did suffer, but she and her family trusted God. Eternity holds all the answers.

The glory of Alysa's healing and recovery is God's. Alysa is a miracle. There isn't anybody who says it wasn't God, and I harbor no doubt for her complete recovery.

Interview with Sylvia Rivers
I fix the church supper twice a month at Northwood Baptist Church. The meal is especially liked by the seniors. There are only about 60 there, so it's a manageable amount of people. We have salad, meat, roll, a vegetable and a dessert. I love doing it because they enjoy it so much.

I was doing the cooking at church that first Wednesday night that Alysa came to thank everyone for his or her prayers. She had only been home for about a month. Everyone rejoiced with tears in his eyes that Alysa had recovered. Alysa always has loved older folks, and it was remarkable and thrilling that she remembered their names. Their hope and faith was demonstrated in the flesh. Praise the Lord!

Interview with Andy Rivers

Alysa's homecoming made our spirits soar. Our prayers had been answered. We remained a little apprehensive, because we didn't know what to expect. Again, we depended on the Lord to handle the therapy, the speech, the memory—everything. She had a long way to go, and we planned to get out of God's way and let him do the work.

A year has passed since September 1997, and today I believe she will have a complete recovery. She has started to bug me and tease me like crazy. She tries to aggravate me—and she succeeds. That's the joking, happy, independent Alysa from before all this happened.

Our faith grew tremendously and we are not afraid to trust God for everything. Physically, things may be hard to handle, but spiritually we remain totally confident. That confidence helps Sylvia and me relate to others in need. Other friends and church members experience tougher times than we did. Now we feel qualified to help them through their difficult times. We know what it's like. We've been there.

In Second Corinthians it says, "God…comforts us in all our troubles, so that we can comfort those in any trouble."

Interview with Dr. Dan Abraham

I visited Alysa several times when she was in Crooked Creek in Grand Blanc. They took great care of her there. How can I make her a little bit better, even for an hour, seemed to be their philosophy. Usually I would go and just sit. Once I tapped her on the shoulder while she was sleeping. Alys? Are you awake? I had asked her. "Yeah, yeah, I'm awake," she said and rolled back over, asleep. She scared me to death! But I had finally heard her voice. It was sweet.

Returning to the hospital, I'd have to give everyone a report.

It would be a miserable day for me—I couldn't get any work done. My replies became automatic as I tried to do my paperwork and read the charts. Alysa was not forgotten at Oakhill.

As she improved, I was aware that she did not exhibit the brain damage we expect after such an illness. Her thinking always showed higher cognitive thought processes. She was quick and could understand sarcasm. She definitely did not want to be babied. I could joke with her and she would smile if something were funny. That is not typical. She has a very good memory of her past—all except her illness. Very few people remember being in ICU. It saddens me that she lost an entire year of her life. I hate that. I feel she was ignored a bit by the profession, and somehow I wanted to make it up to her.

I really don't think any of the doctors did a damn thing for her. Her recovery came from within her family. Her recovery was a gift.

Interview with Sandy Barnes

As I reflect on the impact of Alysa's situation on others, and especially her mother, I see Linda as a living, walking illustration of true Biblical faith as listed in Hebrews 11.

Linda never seemed desperate or desperately pleading for her own desired outcome in Alysa's healing. She did have the desire to see her daughter well, and she believed that our God of the impossible could heal her—if that were his plan. Instead, Linda had a complete trust and peace in God's design.

Linda, aware that God could use Alysa in a state of illness as well as in a state of wellness, prayed for his will and not her own. Linda, with no self-will, let God be God. The centerpiece of Linda's faith remained in the deity of God. Her faith did not attempt to manipulate God into her game plan, but allowed his eternal reasoning.

I don't mean to glorify Linda. Her God is glorified. I praise him that he found someone in this lifetime that could be trusted to display him, his mysterious plans and his peace so beautifully. This picture of faith has purified my own personal faith.

Interview with Brenda Cox

I became joyous when Alysa started to show improvement.

She began to make eye contact, recognize people and re-learn how to swallow. These were all major hurdles. She had not yet spoken.

A gentleman at Linda's parents' church vowed to fast and pray specifically for Alysa's speech. At that time no one had a clue of her abilities. Soon after his commitment Alysa announced, "I want to go to church." One man's mission had made a difference. "Oh ye of little faith."

When my daughter Andrea was four months pregnant, she had a virus that we later discovered went to the baby's brain. Alexandria was born brain damaged. The doctors told us she was deaf, mute and blind. But she is ten months old and she can hear and see. Because of Linda's example of faith, it no longer matters to me what the doctors say. God isn't finished with Alexandria yet; Andrea recalls and claims for herself Linda's example of faith when she visited Alysa in the nursing home.

Linda and Dave taught us about hope. Through their experience we learned not to focus on the negatives and the setbacks. Someday Alexandria will be the person God wants her to be. To reinforce that hope, all I have to do is look at Alysa.

I saw her recently. It's been a year since she left the nursing home. She's doing her own makeup, choosing her own clothing, helping out in the kitchen and re-learning how to drive. I do not question that she will have a normal, God-filled life. And her sense of humor seems wittier than before. She's quite a card.

Interview with Linda Beaudoin

Alysa's healing is a direct result of prayer. Prayer is such a relief. When I turned my kids over to God, I felt a burden lifted. He will watch over them. Now that my children have witnessed this remarkable journey, they have all begun the search for their own spiritual development.

Yes, this is definitely a love story. Ken's for Alysa. Linda's for Alysa. Dave's for Alysa. In the future someday I hope I'll have a little Alysa and a little Kendrick as a result of all that love.

Interview with Ken Komisarz

Alysa need not worry about my salvation anymore. On November 1, 1997, in the morning service at Faith Baptist

Church, I went forward at the invitation at the close of the service. There I confessed my belief in Jesus Christ as the one true God and my own personal Savior. I was baptized that night and both of our families were there to witness.

I don't have any doubt about the future. Even if Alysa doesn't come back all the way, I see us together always. Yeah, I plan to marry her. I don't know when. God's timing will decide when we're ready.

Interview with Carrie Komisarz

Our family became even closer through Alysa's tragedy. Kenny needed our support. I realize how important it is to let people know how you feel about them. I am so thankful for my family.

Interview with Kelly Komisarz

Seeing God work in her life made me want to return to my own faith. I've gotten my confirmation and my first communion. I believe that God kept Alysa alive. Everyone said she should be dead—that her body should have given up many times. I understand what it is to have hope and trust in the Lord.

Interview with Pat Toth

It was at Crooked Creek that Alysa started to improve. The drama of her first words was broadcast to prayer groups throughout the state and beyond.

My daughter Becky and I went out one afternoon. Alysa was sitting in a wheelchair with the beach ball she used to improve eye-hand coordination. Very politely she said, "It's nice to meet you" after I told her who we were. Because her short-term memory eluded her, only seconds later she would ask, "Now who are you again?" We didn't mind telling her a hundred times who we were. Hearing her speak was its own reward.

At first her thoughts and actions were childish. Then she became more willful, which I called her teenage stage, where she wanted to do things her own way.

Pete was one of the ones to help Alysa first learn to walk. He would hold her by the armpits and Becky would move Alysa's feet for her. Everyone got sweaty and spent from the exertion.

"Okay, I want to stand up again," Alysa would say. It was good sweat!

Seeing the Lord restore her is a miracle. Once she is physically and spiritually whole, her life will be a testimony forever. The Lord didn't allow this to happen without a reason. I have already seen a lot of good from this tragedy: the acceptance of Christ by Linda's grandmother, Linda's father's recommitment to the Lord, and Ken and Ken's mother's salvation, to name only a few. Who knows what other seeds have been planted in the hundreds of people who came in touch with Linda and Dave.

Their faith can be an example for our family as we face our own adventure. No matter what the Lord calls me to go through, he'll be here lifting me up—just as he was for them. We believe that the Lord wants us to leave this area and go somewhere else. And that somewhere is Nashville, Tennessee. We are trusting God's call for our new location. The words in Steve Green's song "The Plan" mirror our viewpoint. We don't need to know God's plan for us. We just follow him wherever he leads and do whatever he asks us to do.

I have given teas as an outreach in a local nursing home, have had new member teas in my home to welcome people to the church, and have hosted elaborate ladies' teas with special music and an inspirational speaker at Faith Baptist Church. Perhaps over a cup of tea in Nashville, Tennessee, the story of Alysa and her family of faith will steep in a needy vessel.

Interview with Cindy Schmidler

Alysa's testimony when she is totally well will be amazing! She went into the coma loving God and she remembered that love from the depths of her being. It is so important to teach our children the love of the Lord. It is the greatest gift that we can give them.

Linda was willing to allow God to use her and her daughter to reach others for Christ. Through her obedience and faith he will continue to bless them. Love is about relationships: a mother and a daughter, a husband and a wife, best friends, God with his children.

I'm blessed to have known them and to have seen this miracle first hand. I can tell others about God's love. I can say to people, let me tell you about my friend Linda. God takes us through suffering in our lives so we can trust in him. Through suffering we can find comfort in him. Then we have his ability to comfort others. Paul in Second Corinthians says "...God...who comforts us in all our troubles, so that we can comfort those in any trouble with the comfort we ourselves have received from God."

Linda and I will always be best friends. I can call her at any moment and know that she will get on her knees and be my prayer warrior. What more can you ask for in a friend?

Interview with Steve Moffett

My heart rejoiced when Alysa left the nursing home for an overnight and I went to see her. She kissed Ken and her dad and said when asked, "Yeah, I know Steve." Linda and Dave brought her to our house for a cookout in July of '97. She was in a wheelchair and everyone felt sorry for her. Linda protested. "No. No. She's much better. You have no idea how bad she was."

I do know. I know, too, that God answers prayers. Alysa has come through the tunnel to the other side. She may never be exactly the same Alysa as before, but she'll have a happy, productive life. She'll be a living testimony to the rest of us. Hebrews 11:1 tells us, "Faith is being sure of what we hope for and certain of what we do not see."

AUTHOR'S NOTE

Many people casually refer to luck, coincidence, good fortune and being in the right place at the right time. Those explanations are the words of man. There is one who controls every aspect of our lives and that is the Lord. He decides what person we will meet by "chance" on any given day. He is totally in charge of our everyday happenings. Divine providence directs our course on this earth.

It was not by chance that we attended Faith Baptist Church one morning and met John and Cindy Schmidler. It was not fate that prompted them to later introduce us to Linda and Dave Conselyea. It was not coincidental that I had always planned to write a book. God orchestrated each step of the way. In turn we are to give him credit for his guidance and thanksgiving for his showering of blessings.

The Conselyeas never doubted who was in control of their daughter. They recognized God's love for them and his power to work miracles. They never asked "Why me, Lord?" because the simple answer was "Why not?" We often think we are exempt from pain and suffering. When there's a crook in our path or when life deals us a blow, we are surprised. Actually we are being tested to see how we fare. Do we fall apart and blame God or trust God and await the eternal explanation for our pain? The story of Alysa Conselyea and her family's perseverance will remain as an

260

example of how each one of us can react with faith in God's perfect plan.

The best thing about this book is that it doesn't end on this page. Alysa is a thriving, remarkable, determined young woman who is progressing daily. Her own hopes and dreams are within her grasp. We wish her God's continued blessings.

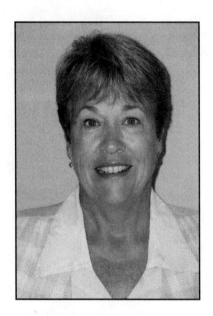

KATHY EVERNHAM

Kathy Evernham, a free-lance humorist writer, has written her first serious book. Her life experiences and resident locations in six different states continue to lend her subject matter. She lived in the Detroit area when she became deeply touched by Alysa's story.

Now a Daytona Beach, Florida resident with summers in the Grand Traverse Michigan area, she resides with her pilot husband, Tom.

She lists being a stained glass artist, a painter and an avid tennis player as her favorite pastimes, but enjoying her grand-children takes first place.